Praise for *From Eating Disorders to Fully Live*

"This unique exploration of adolescent onset eating disorders is not about therapy or treatment; it's about narrative and journey. From two different generations, Melissa and Alayna, explore universal topics, one's that crystallize and threaten when an eating disorder takes hold. They connect and reflect about their personal journeys to emotional growth and transcendence. Their voices are unique, yet the vulnerabilities they share and challenges they face are not only at the core of the recovery process but perhaps, universal to successfully navigating adult development. The result is informative and inspirational."

Kim McCallum MD; Psychiatrist, Author, Advocate Founder McCallum Place Eating Disorders Treatment Centers, CEDS, Former member, Board of Directors National Eating Disorders Association and of International Association of Eating Disorders Professionals, Co-Founder, Missouri Eating Disorders Association

"Searching for an understanding to unlock the prison of fear and conditioning that the world creates in us, Alayna and Melissa share their different perspectives on universal topics around eating disorders. Through these testimonies, we discern the progress that has been made in mental health but also how much more there is to learn. Placing the narrative of these two women side by side, the book gives each story a new perspective. Alayna is young, at the start of her adult life with childhood still fresh in her memory. Melissa is a mother with a career in business and a host of life achievements and milestones to look back on.

As you move between the two stories, something remarkable happens. In this dialogue between the generations, we understand so much of the ever-changing challenge in becoming a whole person; integrating the person you were, the person you are and the person you want to be and all the miraculous transitions that will happen in between. In this book we see how a full life is truly more than the sum of its parts.

Like any mental struggle, there are many roads into eating disorders and many roads out. Alayna and Melissa are not interested in simplistic solutions. They understand that no one knows exactly what you need and there is no "playbook" for the triggers of eating disorders. But they want you to know you are not alone and in this uniting of the generations, they demonstrate the essence of true community, transforming "self-help" into the "together-help" that it should always be.

In this book you will not find prescriptive answers, or expert advice. In reading this book you will find something much more urgently needed: you will find kinship, acceptance and, above all, hope."

Nigel C Lester MD, Psychiatrist
Director of Mental Health, PALM Health
Professor, Anthropedia Foundation
St Louis MO

Full

Overcoming our Eating Disorders to Fully Live

ALAYNA J. BURKE AND MELISSA L. KELLEY

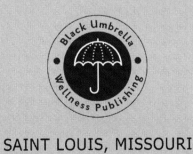

SAINT LOUIS, MISSOURI

Copyright © 2022 by Black Umbrella Wellness Publishing, LLC
Full: Overcoming our Eating Disorders to Fully Live

All rights reserved. No part of this book may be reproduced or transmitted in any form or by any means without written permission of the authors or publishers. BlackUmbrellaWellness@gmail.com

Paperback ISBN: 979-8-9867840-0-7
eBook ISBN: 979-8-9867840-1-4

Printed in the United States of America
Published in the United States of America

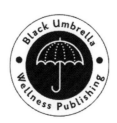

For my parents, Tom and Patty Burke, for putting up with my shit for so long without hesitation

—Alayna

In honor of my beautiful mother, Barbara Kelley, for loving me through the chaos and terror of an eating disorder while raising five other children

—Melissa

Contents

Preface x

Part 1: Our Stories...1

Alayna...3
Melissa 19

Part 2: Underlying Issues . . .
It's Never Really about the Food...................................39

Chapter 1: Trauma..41
Chapter 2: Fear of Growing Up 61
Chapter 3: Body Image...76
Chapter 4: Thin or Small Equals.............................89
Chapter 5: Be a Lady...99
Chapter 6: Shame 113
Chapter 7: Perfectionism 132
Chapter 8: Control 146
Chapter 9: Comparison 156
Chapter 10: Glamorizing Being Sick......................165
Chapter 11: Healthy Addictions 176
Chapter 12: Triggers..185

Part 3: Guideposts...193

Personal Practices that Can Help.........................195
A Letter to the Reader 214
Book Club Study Questions.................................220
Recommendations from Our Bookshelves..........................221

Acknowledgments 223
About the Authors 227

Listen Closely, What Do You See?

Noise ushers in the mirage
The illusion of water to your thirsty soul
The image of perfection is cast
In the distance, colorful, shimmery, transparent

Loud and bright
Words that cut
Pictures that lie
Sounds that pierce
Grasping, chasing, longing
Just one more
Just one less

When you close your eyes, do you hear her?
When you hear her voice, do you see her?

She brings you home with lights dancing on your eyelids
The breath going in
The shoulders going down
She's the watcher
She's the listener
She's home
She's been waiting for you

~ Melissa Kelley

Preface

We're from different generations. Melissa was born in 1968, Alayna in the early 2000s. Melissa went to high school with Alayna's parents, and they remain friends today. When Alayna decided to write a book about her eating disorder experience and recovery, Melissa jumped at the chance to join her, since she'd started and stopped her own memoir of this experience many times.

We aren't clinicians, and this book isn't intended to be prescriptive. We tell our stories for girls and women struggling with eating disorders. We tell our stories to provide hope for a fuller life—a life free of the loneliness and despair of an eating disorder. We represent two very different generations and hope to reach as many readers as we can. And although Alayna grew up thirty years after Melissa, and children today are growing up decades after Alayna, much pressure remains for women's bodies to reflect an ever-changing ideal. This pressure begins early in life and the message pervades all forms of media.

Jane Fonda, the Academy Award-winning actress who launched the home fitness revolution with her workout videos in the 1980s, battled bulimia for decades. In her 2011 interview with *Harper's Bazaar,* she begins her story with, "I was raised in the '50s. I was taught by my father [actor Henry Fonda] that how I looked was all that mattered, frankly. He was a good man, and I was mad for him, but he sent messages to me that fathers shouldn't send: unless you look perfect, you're not going to be loved."

Every generation brings about different versions of the same problem. In Melissa's youth, the diet and home fitness industries soared, and diet product commercials were as ubiquitous as the pharmaceutical advertisements of the 2010s and 2020s. Women were shamelessly graded on their appearance, as in the 1979 film titled *10*, referencing the protagonist's "perfect woman." Most notably, this was a time when mental health wasn't openly discussed and when mental illness was shamed.

In the 1972 US presidential election, George McGovern chose Missouri Senator Tom Eagleton as his running mate against Richard Nixon and Spiro Agnew. Within days of this announcement, it was discovered that in the 1960s, Senator Eagleton had undergone electroshock therapy during three hospitalizations for depression. Eighteen days into their campaign, and under tremendous pressure from the Democratic Party, Senator Eagleton withdrew his candidacy.

When Alayna was growing up in the 2000s and 2010s, mental health, while arguably still stigmatized, was a much more mainstream topic as the world reeled from the aftermath of the 9/11 terrorist attack on the United States. Personal computers and smartphones were woven into the fabric of her reality at a young age, and she grew up as part of the social media generation in which every moment could be captured and shared instantly, and people incessantly posted filtered pictures of themselves and others at their most beautiful and happiest.

In this current environment, with constant pressure to present social media post-worthy bodies and faces, Alayna needed immense courage and fortitude to let go of her eating disorder behavior in only two years (supported by outpatient treatment).

Melissa's eating disorder was active for six years between the ages of sixteen and twenty-one, during which time she was hospitalized three times and supported by intensive outpatient programs. In response to trauma, Melissa's eating disorder took on a new form in her thirties and was managed through outpatient treatment. It has been over thirty years since her last hospitalization, and in addition to information about those active years, she shares how her eating disorder thoughts and tendencies have manifested throughout her adulthood and the strategies she uses to keep those behaviors at bay.

Both of us reference our active eating disorder years as a period during which we sat on the sidelines of life. We're so grateful to have found our way back to fully living our lives—lives filled with experiences that bring both good and bad emotions, love and loss, despair and triumph.

It's our intention that this book bring hope, inspiration, and motivation to anyone who has stepped into the depths of an eating disorder. You're likely sensitive, empathetic, perfectionistic, or just plain scared that the overwhelm this world brings to *everyone* is too much for you. We've been there, and we have moments that tug at us to step aside once more. And we choose to be full. Join us.

Part 1: Our Stories

Alayna

From the outside, my childhood was pretty idyllic. I was born three years after my brother Nathan. I grew up with the support of two parents (who were high school sweethearts), and they are still married today. As a family, we grew up with a Catholic education, we went on adventurous vacations, we played every sport you can think of, and we spent time with our neighbors and friends as much as we could. The four of us were fun-loving and hardworking. However, because I was always comfortable, I felt that I couldn't ever express my struggles because others had it worse. In other words, I told myself complaining made me a stuck-up, privileged girl.

My earliest memory of hating my body is of going to the doctor for my annual checkup at about ten years old. I hadn't grown into my body yet, so naturally I was a little chubby. But I'd never thought twice about my size until the doctor showed me my growth chart, took a deep breath, and told me I might want to "lay off the snacks." Little did that doctor know that my perfectionist self would use that as motivation for the next seven years to reject my body. You can probably guess what I gave up for Lent that year: snacks. This is merely one story of many that built up to my anxiety, depression, and eating disorder.

If you know me, you know that once I set my mind on a goal, there's no doubt that I'm going to absolutely annihilate it. One of my obsessions at that age was tumbling. My best friend Emily did gymnastics and, at ten years old, I thought she was the coolest person because of it. So, soon enough, I was practicing handstands and backbend kickovers until I could feel my brain pulsing in my skull. I learned some cool tricks eventually, but something else came with my hard work: weight loss. That wasn't my goal, but when I came back to school after that summer, I heard a girl whispering at the lunch table behind me: "Guys, Alayna looks so much better now that she's tiny." No more chubby phase, I guess. For the rest of my preteen and teenage years, I took pride in the summer that I lost weight, and I'd often point it out when looking through old pictures just to feel that reassurance that I accomplished a great feat. However, there'd always be a voice in the back of my head saying, "Never let yourself get chubby again." Losing weight gave me approval, pride, and attention.

Until about fifteen years old, I was oblivious to the fact that everyone had internal struggles. I had normal insecurities, and I compared myself to my best friends all the time, but I never knew that those same best friends had their own issues. Of course, today it seems like everyone is aware of the importance of mental health, but in the early 2000s, that stuff was more of a whisper. That's why my classmates and I held our breaths and widened our eyes when teachers started giving brutal presentations on the effects of depression, alcohol, drugs, sex, you name it. *Yikes. Shove those terrible things into the back of your mind, Alayna. You won't ever need to worry about those,* I told myself.

I've mentioned how I was (and definitely still am) a perfectionist. I was that toddler who got upset when others didn't put the crayons back in the box in rainbow order. In preschool, while other kids were playing at recess, I cleaned the rocks out of the play shed. This obsession cost me one day when a boy in my preschool class didn't want the shed to be clean. I shoveled the rocks out of the shed, and he threw them back in. So, I slapped his arm. "WHHAAAA. Ouch, Alayna!" he said, then ran to tell the teacher. I only remember that because it was one of the only times I ever got in trouble, and of course it was for cleaning.

I was the quiet kind of perfectionist: the girl who worked her ass off in silence just to sneak up on everyone and win when it mattered most. That was my goal, to win. Everything was a competition. Be the smartest, funniest, most athletic, loudest, quietest, coolest, happiest, friendliest, most likable person in any room. I think it's safe to say this attitude was the root of my later struggles because being the best at everything simply isn't realistic. I was even competitive in my friendships, and I sometimes found it hard to be happy for my friends' accomplishments. Of course, I loved all of my friends growing up, but I always felt like I was lacking deep connections. I saw the friends on TV and social media that told each other everything, and I craved that closeness.

I desired deeper friendships at a very young age. But I had trouble finding friends who were comfortable with serious conversations, and continually felt like I was missing something. Even within my family I felt that same craving for connection, but it seemed like I was the only one who wanted to talk about my deepest feelings and thoughts. I thank God for my spiritual life because it often gave me the connection I needed. I started taking my faith seriously around eighth grade, and I'll forever be thankful that I set a strong spiritual foundation before I went off to high school.

I never liked following the crowd, so I chose a high school where I knew only a few people. I was a friendly girl, genuinely excited to meet new people, but each day at school I felt socially rejected. My first day, I recognized a girl from mutual friends on social media and introduced myself. Here's how it went.

Me: "Hi! I'm Alayna. Are you friends with [my friend]? You look familiar."

Girl: *crinkles eyebrows and walks away*

Not a great first interaction in my opinion, but I didn't let it get to me. *Bitches will be bitches*, I thought. Rejection got old, though. The day I got fed up was when I sat down in the library with some girls who were in my classes.

I said, "Hi," went to the bathroom, and came back to find my stuff sitting alone at the table. They'd all moved to a different table and stared at me and laughed as I began working on my homework alone. It sounds like a movie, right? Instead of brushing it off, this time I took it personally, assuming there was something wrong with me that made these girls dislike me.

The rest of my first semester of high school consisted of me trying to be as invisible as possible. I stopped craving deep connections. School was just a place for me to learn and get straight As, nothing else. My family knew I wasn't happy, and one night I finally told them I wanted to transfer to a school where a lot of my grade school friends were. I'm beyond grateful for how supportive my family was in my decision and how much they helped me with the transition. A new school would give me a new chance at making connections . . . or so I thought.

Don't get me wrong, I loved my new school and the girls there. It really was a fresh start, and I genuinely felt welcomed. But past rejections left scars, and I soon felt the pressures of popularity. My brother had always been the partier and social butterfly, and now I was the one being exposed to parties, drinking, and boys. I just wanted to have a good time, but each time I drank or went to a party, I'd end my night crying in the bathroom. Ironically, my loneliest moments were those in big crowds. But I didn't allow myself to admit that I was struggling because I felt like I should be happy after my family had gone through the hassle of transferring me. Sometimes people would find me in the bathrooms crying, but I told them I was just tired. I figured nobody wanted to hear a sob story that wasn't even worth sobbing over.

There came a point where I felt so disconnected from my friends that I became afraid of social interaction. One day, I faked a stomachache instead of going to a concert, and that one choice spiraled into a series of turning down my friends' invitations. I can't blame them for not seeing my behavior as a cry for help because they had their own lives to figure out, and I tend to be a hard case to open when I'm upset. However, I wanted so badly for someone to recognize my pain without having to tell them.

My parents and I noticed a real problem when I started having nightmares and anxiety attacks. My nightmares always involved being abandoned by my friends without knowing why. I loved volleyball at the time, but even at tournaments I'd run off the court in the middle of the game with a panic attack. To say I was humiliated would be an understatement. If you've never had a panic attack, it feels like you're about to die, and you can't do anything to stop it. Your chest heats up, your heart starts skipping beats, and your hands shake. You want to pull your hair out in a combination of anger, sadness, and fear.

Soon enough I was having panic attacks every morning before school. One day I'll never forget was when my mom drove me to school because I was too humiliated to ride in my carpool with two girls I'd known since kindergarten. Once we turned into the parking lot, I started screaming and crying. The thought of focusing on school and facing social pressure was torture. My friends across the parking lot saw me sitting in my mom's car with tears streaming down my face, so I slid down slowly in my seat. My poor mom had no idea how to handle this. There was no way I could make it through the school day, so she angrily drove me back home and called my pediatrician. I felt nothing but anger toward my mom for thinking this was a medical issue.

Before I knew it, I was paired with a therapist. Unfortunately, one of the outlets I turned to was cutting myself to make the pain real. After the first time I cut my wrist, I kept it a secret until I couldn't bear the thought of lying to my family. I walked up to my dad one morning before school and said, "I don't know why I did this," showing him my wrist. Tears slid down my cheeks, but I was too exhausted to show any further emotion. That was the first time in my life I'd ever seen my dad cry. I was expecting an outburst from him, but the love he gave me in that moment is the love I hope I can give my kids in the future. From then on, it was okay to tell my dad what I was feeling.

Therapy was a nightmare. Picture this: a pale, tired, stubborn teenage girl sitting on a couch with her arms folded, staring into space. I was doing it for my parents, not myself. I'd be assigned homework such as, "Make plans with an old friend one time this month." It never happened.

Here's where food came into play. Since I felt out of control and needed a distraction, I turned to restricting my food. But this had to be an ultimate secret. I became vegan as an excuse to eat less, but I told everyone it was, "for the environment and my health." Restricting was my new favorite game to play. I kept a page of notes on my phone where I'd record everything I ate in a day, and it had to be five items or fewer. I weighed myself at least twice a day to make sure I was getting smaller. And the most isolating thing I did was leave my food at home, so I could study instead of sitting with people at lunch.

My mom, being the caretaker she naturally is, noticed the changes I was making and finally confronted me about it. I claimed I just wanted to eat healthier, but even I knew that was a lie. The truth was that if I looked sick then I wouldn't have to explain to people how I was feeling inside—they'd be able to see the hurt on the outside.

At this point, I'd quit volleyball and my job at an ice cream shop because I couldn't keep up mentally or physically. Therapy was going okay, but my therapist diagnosed me with anxiety and depression with OCD tendencies related to eating and exercise. Ouch. I felt like a problem. Sitting in the waiting room for therapy with other kids who had obvious emotional and behavioral issues wasn't a great feeling. *Why can't I help myself? This is pathetic.*

Since things weren't getting better, it was time to talk about medication. I'll never forget the day I went to my pediatrician. She weighed me, which gave me something to focus on, and sat me down to go over what I'd been going through. The moment she looked at my growth chart and saw a dramatic drop in weight, she said something no one had asked me yet: "Please tell me what's going on." Her eyes were filled with tears, and I was beyond confused because all she did was see I'd lost weight. But something about that look in her eyes made me feel like she saw right through me, so I told her how I'd been struggling with social anxiety, depression, and restricting my food. She was the best listener.

After I'd finished, she went on to tell my mom—and me—that her own daughter had an eating disorder. Those two words made my throat close up. *No, that's not me. Why would she say that?* She knew exactly where I was headed, and she said she was going to do everything she could to make sure I didn't spiral. I hated her at that moment because she'd just exposed me for something no one had the nerve to bring up. She suggested that I take an anxiety medication and see a psychiatrist. They also decided that it was time for a new therapist that specialized in eating disorders. Her next objective was to find me a dietitian, and of course my mom was scribbling down names as fast as she could so she could go home and research every professional who could hopefully fix me.

My life became centered around appointments. Therapist, psychiatrist, dietitian, and now group therapy, too. Some I dreaded, and some I relied on. But I still couldn't wrap my head around the fact that I was in serious danger. Was it all in my head? Were these doctors against me?

I was starting my junior year of high school. I took easier classes in order to focus on getting better, so I gained a lot of free time. I was obsessed with exercise, but I'd finally found a healthy coping mechanism . . . yoga. I'll go into more detail about this later, but in a nutshell, yoga was often the only way I could separate my good thoughts from my eating disorder thoughts.

Another thing that filled my time was a brand-new sport: cross-country. I joined cross-country on the second day of tryouts simply because of a vivid dream I'd had. I dreamed that I was running on the team and laughing and smiling the entire time. This might not seem significant, but for some reason it woke me up at 3:00 a.m. and made my heart pound because it made me feel so happy.

Joining cross-country was the best decision I made in high school because it reminded me how much I enjoyed being around people and doing the things I loved. Running burns a lot of calories, and that was attractive to me, but it was also another way to get me unstuck. As soon as the starting gun went off at races, my mind would go blank, and I'd have a little over twenty minutes of total escape from thoughts of my eating disorder and depression. I even learned that I was pretty darn fast, too!

The downside of cross-country, however, was that it boosted the rate at which I lost weight, and I loved it. Running is extremely addictive, and I was good at it, so when my dietitian told me I should consider quitting in order to gain weight, I was furious. This woman really wanted to take away the one thing that I thought was getting me to a better place? Where was the proof that I was unhealthy? I was fine!

But I was far from fine. In fact, I started to notice the physical signs of starvation at their worst. My hair began to fall out in clumps, I couldn't stand up without my vision going black. I got my first cavity ever, and I got an EKG that showed my heart rate was about as low as an Olympic athlete's.

Each time I noticed the signs, I'd have mixed feelings of accomplishment and fear. Accomplishment because it meant that maybe other people could finally see my pain, and fear because I knew eating disorders were fatal. I became obsessed with watching YouTube videos about girls sharing their eating disorder stories, and I'd panic each time because they all ended up hospitalized. Although it scared me, I was so consumed by that lifestyle that I told myself I was okay with getting that sick. *I'm not that bad yet.*

The worst parts of my eating disorder were the supplement drinks and meal plans because it meant control was ripped out of my hands. My dietitian required me to drink an Ensure Plus once a day and would write out meal plans so that I got more than enough of each food group. My mom was a nurse, so of course she took these meal plans seriously and became my personal cook. On Thanksgiving, she made my plate. She packed my lunch every day. And I'll never forget how she sat in my room until I finished my Ensure every single night. That drink was a huge threat to my eating disorder, so each night when I finished it, I was moving one step closer to conquering my eating disorder. It didn't go down without a fight, though. One night I was so angry about having to drink that stupid weight-gain drink that I threw the bottle at my mom. She didn't even flinch or get mad; she just sat there until I calmed down and accepted that I had to drink it.

Appointments got depressing because both my therapist and dietitian started exposing me to the idea of inpatient treatment. They said that at the rate I was dropping weight, it was extremely likely that I'd need to be admitted. I didn't know squat about eating disorder treatment. My mom did her research and knew that inpatient treatment wasn't for me. I'm a very independent person, and my mom felt that I wouldn't get much independence in treatment.

She said, "Someone would have to go to the bathroom with you to make sure you don't throw up, and they'll serve you all your meals and require you to finish." Deep down I knew the message she was communicating: she didn't want her baby girl to be sent away. I began to understand her point of view. My biggest fear about inpatient treatment was that I'd be surrounded by other girls with the same toxic mindset as me. I was told, however, by my dietician and therapist that treatment would be necessary. This is when things started to change for the good.

In December, they gave me three weeks to consistently gain weight, or I'd be sent to treatment in Tulsa,

Oklahoma, which was almost a six-hour drive from home. It was suddenly real. I started to think about the things I'd be missing. I'd just met a solid group of friends, I'd just started dating my first boyfriend, I'd just finished an awesome sports season, and I was doing great academically. But the biggest factor was that I wouldn't have my family. They had kept me going this whole time, so how could I just ditch them? My parents didn't show how upset they were that I might be sent away soon—they just kept quietly doing everything they could to give me a normal life.

We went on a ski trip between Christmas and New Year's. My dietitian understood that skiing burns a lot of calories, so she gave me some slack on how much weight I had to gain by the time I came back. However, going out of town didn't mean no Ensure, and it sure as hell didn't mean I could restrict. I didn't think of it this way, but my mom saw it as my last family vacation before treatment.

The way my family sacrificed their time for me on that vacation was unbelievable. If they wanted to go on one more ski run, it would have to wait until after a full lunch. They'd sit with me and wait until I'd finished every bite of each meal. I hadn't told any of my friends about the threat of treatment, and only one friend, Ellen, knew about the eating disorder. Ellen's simple act of FaceTiming with me each night on vacation kept me attached to reality. She made me laugh until my cheeks ached, and I couldn't imagine being stripped away from laughter and friendship.

My favorite moment from the ski trip was when I got my Ensure out of the fridge one night and stared at it with a blank look on my face for about five minutes. *Fuck this drink. I don't need it.* Nathan noticed what was happening and got up off the couch, walked to the fridge, grabbed an Ensure, and chugged it. *WHAT?! How did he do that without freaking out?* It showed me that this one drink wasn't going to kill me and I stopped fighting it so hard. Big brother always knew how to teach me by example.

We got home the next week. I'd been enjoying small moments of life without realizing how much better I was doing. What I didn't know then was that while I was on vacation, my dietitian and therapist had met for lunch and discussed that inpatient was my only option. They thought I was too far gone. But, when my mom and I went to my next appointments, even though I'd gained only about half a pound, my new mindset was a shock to them both. And they let me stay home.

The fight wasn't over yet. Since I'd proven I could continue outpatient treatment, I'd have to stick with it. Soon I realized that choosing to recover would be a daily choice, often a more-than-once-a-day choice. I wish I could say I only went up from there, but healing isn't linear. Let that sink in. Healing. Isn't. Linear. I'd take two steps forward and one step back, but they were monumental steps nonetheless.

In these next chapters, I want to share as much as I can about what I learned that helped me recover. These are all tools I still use daily because my eating disorder holds a spot in my head no matter what. I just have to remember how my eating disorder stole my life.

I like to be hopeful. So, what's Alayna's life like without her eating disorder in control? First of all, I LOVE being social, but I also still have a lot of alone time. I know what balance is and how to find it. I'm quite mentally tough now, meaning I don't take things too personally because I know my worth lies in more than what people think of me. I have more good days than bad because when I have a bad day I know I just have to push on. I make bad decisions sometimes, but I don't regret them, and I own up to them out loud.

I often think about my future and all the mysteries it holds. I see God in my own creative ways. I'm vulnerable whenever I get the chance to be. If someone asks me to share my story, of course I get nervous, but I seize the opportunity to impact others. I'm independent, and I don't rely as much on my parents. I'm surrounded by close friends who know my story and confront me when they see my old habits surfacing.

I still struggle with food sometimes, but my body, mind, and spirit have built up the knowledge of how shitty it feels to be hungry and won't let me restrict myself. I found my love for fitness again, and it's rooted in finding my strongest self, not my thinnest self.

Most importantly, I'm still the same person. I simply know my worth and am proud of who I am. I don't reject my eating disorder self. I forgive her. In the next chapters,

I want to give you hope. Hope for your own recovery or for someone else's recovery. I know I'm a teenager, but if anything, I believe that qualifies me even more than most to provide tips for living fully in modern society.

Melissa

Poker

The beginning returns to me in flashes.

I'm standing next to my parents' bed in front of the gilded full-length mirror. I'm six years old, and I'm wearing my Catholic school uniform—a plaid jumper over a white blouse. Brown hair springs from the widow's peak on my forehead, surrounds my face, and falls to my shoulders. On the other side of the big bed, the black-and-white TV plays the theme to *Gilligan's Island.* I hear it, but my eyes are fixed on the mirror. As I study the reflection of my small frame, fear shoots through me.

That's me. I'm big.

I seemed to take up so much space.

I won't be able to disappear anymore if I'm big.

When I got scared or lonely, I believed that I could disappear. I did this a lot in Mrs. Helweg's first-grade classroom. I had horrible separation anxiety, and I cried every day when I was dropped off at school. I hated being away from my mother. I never felt safe in that big classroom. I'd solved that by learning how to disappear. I'd just close my eyes and think myself little.

In my mind, I could get smaller and smaller until no one could see me. But now this! I was big, and I was petrified.

If this kept up, I wouldn't be able to disappear anymore. I couldn't imagine what would happen then.

We're gathered around the television in the family room. I'm eight years old and my three sisters and I are sprinkled among the couches and floor as mom nurses our new baby brother. We're watching the 1976 Olympic gymnastics competition, and I'm mesmerized by the bodies of these girls with interesting names from places I don't know. Nadia and Olga are the stars. My sister Amy and I pretend we're them as we practice our Olympic floor routines in the front room that doesn't yet have furniture.

Those girls bend and fly, then abruptly stop, then turn and fly again. They're older than me, and their legs look long and seem to connect directly to their rib cages. I can count their ribs. On the uneven bars, Nadia scores the first perfect 10.0 in Olympic history, then goes on to do so six more times. At the end of each routine, she stands with her feet together, her rib cage protruding, her back a letter C. She smiles at the judges, waves to the crowd, and every cell of my being takes note—this is what perfect looks like.

I'm in the school nurse's office on my first day back since being hospitalized for pneumonia. I'm eleven years old, a sixth-grader, and I weigh sixty-three pounds, almost twenty pounds lighter than the average eleven-year-old. Mrs. McCuddy, my band teacher, smiles as she enters the room, so happy to see me after my two weeks away. She puts her hands on my shoulders, and says, "You've lost so much weight!" Then, to the nurse, "Maybe I need to get sick so I can finally lose this weight!"

"Girls, girls! Come in here. I want you to watch this," Mom shouts from the other room.

The living room now has furniture, and a master suite has been added, along with another baby sister. I rush into Mom and Dad's bedroom and see Mom watching a movie on the small TV next to the new bathroom. It's called *The Best Little Girl in the World.*

My only real memory of the movie was seeing the anorexic girl's skeletal body when her sister walked in on her changing clothes. So many bones. So much discipline. So much control. I wanted to be like her. After all, she was the best little girl in the world.

Cards in a poker hand, these four events nestled comfortably with my ace in the hole—a sensitive, approval-seeking person-ality. A royal flush. The perfect hand. For an eating disorder.

Not-So-Sweet Sixteen

I'd just thrown up my after-school snack. There was proba-bly ice cream involved, as that was the easiest thing to throw up in the beginning. I ran out the door to meet dad in the driveway—we were going driving! I'd just started my junior year of high school and was one of the youngest in the class, ergo one of the last to drive.

High school had started out great.

"Just be nice to everyone, Missy," my elderly neighbor said as I bounced nervously in her driveway the evening before my first day.

That resonated deep within me and, as a people pleaser, it was right up my alley. I made it my mission to smile and greet everyone I passed in the halls. It seemed I was happy all the time during freshman year. I was quite popular and was even elected to the homecoming court in the spring. I peaked early, as they say.

Sophomore year proved to be a much bigger challenge for me as alcohol joined the ranks among the popular. My parents were very strict about alcohol and proud of the Kelley family name. "Remember you're a Kelley Girl," was the last thing my dad said to us every time we left the house. The message was 50% "Rah-Rah, you're special and don't you forget it," and 50% "Don't you dare disgrace us and don't think for a second I won't find out about it if you do." Additionally, I played sports—volleyball, basketball, track—and at the start of each season, we committed to the team and ourselves that we wouldn't drink alcohol or use drugs.

By the time junior year rolled around, my popularity had taken a nosedive. I was no longer cool because I didn't drink, and my presence at social outings just made the drinkers feel guilty and paranoid. My self-esteem had plummeted, and smiling and greeting people in the hall didn't do the trick anymore.

I spat out the toothpaste and checked my eyes in the mirror. A little bloodshot but sunglasses would do the trick. I ran out the door and jumped into the latest of Dad's Lincoln Continentals with the license plate "AFL-CIO." He was the president of the governing body for all the unions in the St. Louis metropolitan area, and his appearance fit the stereotype perfectly. He was overweight, he wore a trench coat in the rain, and he drove a luxury sedan.

Driving with Dad was always a treat. He was an intimidating man, large and loud, but he somehow had the patience to teach us all how to drive. I was his third student, and, naturally, was being compared to my older sisters' skills at the same point in their training. He said I was the best. I've no doubt he said that to each one of us!

It was a sunny afternoon, and we'd been practicing for a couple months. I had my permit and must have been driving especially well that day because Dad spontaneously suggested that we go take the test.

"Today? Right now?" I stuttered, feeling a combination of excitement and anxiety. This wasn't the plan, but Dad thought I was ready, and I really wanted my license.

I don't remember much about taking the test, other than that I got The Lady. She was infamous. She was like a character in a funny movie who wasn't funny at all, yet so bizarre that you had no other way to process her presence but to laugh. She wasn't unlike Ben Stein in the 1986 movie *Ferris Bueller's Day Off,* whose monotone chant, "Anyone...anyone...George Washington," made him famous.

The Lady was small with short reddish-brown hair. I saw only the side of her face as she sat in the car, stared out the windshield, and barked her commands in a monotone, staccato voice that was highly unnerving and somewhat inhuman. "WHEN . . . IT . . . IS . . . SAFE . . . TO . . . DO . . . SO . . . TURN . . . RIGHT."

Perhaps she was frightened into this state from years of testing new drivers. On that beautiful September afternoon, I added my name to the list of The Lady's victims. I failed the driving test.

My father felt horrible. He wasn't disappointed in me; he was disappointed in himself for suggesting I take the test. His fantasy was that we would walk into the house at dinnertime and surprise everyone with the news that I was officially A Driver. He apologized profusely and told me it was his fault; that he should have known I wasn't ready. He said it would be our secret. He wouldn't tell any of my sisters, or even my mother. No harm, no foul. Just forget it ever happened.

As they say, the cover-up is usually worse than the crime, and that definitely applied here. I failed the driving test. Maybe I wasn't ready; maybe I was, but The Lady scared me silly. By keeping this our little secret, Dad was trying to spare my feelings and save me from embarrassment. Instead, I internalized this failure, and it fed my shame. Failing the driving test was so shameful that we couldn't speak of it, not even to family. Shame fed my eating disorder.

The Plan

It was a nondescript weekday afternoon in October. I'd passed the driving test, it was volleyball season, and I'd been throwing up my food for months. I was folding one of the perpetual loads of laundry (that were a permanent fixture on the family room floor) in front of the TV, which was always on. Mom was in the kitchen with Bobbie Nolan, her best friend.

The thing I hated most about laundry duty was putting the clean clothes away. On one of my trips back from the bedrooms to the family room, I said, "Mom, I've been throwing up a lot lately."

"What do you mean?" She looked at me with a confused expression.

"After I eat, I throw up."

"Why?" She asked.

"I can't help it," I lied. "When I'm full, I throw up."

"Then don't eat so much," she said.

"OK." *Well, that was easy.*

It's become evident to me that we do very few things by accident, and I'm certain it was no accident that I waited to tell my mother about my problem until there was air cover. Bobbie Nolan would be the voice of reason, and more importantly, she'd be a great support to my mom over the next few months as we ventured into a whole new world.

I don't believe I ever told my parents that I was throwing up to avoid getting fat, or even that I was doing it on purpose. Within a week or so of dropping the bomb on Mom, there was a meeting with the pediatrician. After that appointment, we implemented The Plan.

The Plan was that I'd never be alone. I wouldn't go into a bathroom stall alone. At home or at school, someone would be assigned to follow my every move. Dad talked to the parents of a few of my girlfriends to make sure they were on board with their children being my monitors, and from that point forward, I was watched. Every waking moment.

The Plan didn't work. In fact, I remember drinking a milkshake with one of my monitors and then vomiting it back into the cup as I pretended to take more sips. I thought this was brilliant. I was so skilled at throwing up ice cream that I could do it right in front of people and they couldn't tell. Now, *that* was being in control.

28 Days

I entered the hospital at the beginning of November 1984, the year I turned sixteen. This was my choice. In fact, I think my parents would have preferred that we just stick with The Plan. I'd met with Dr. Larocca, who was the world-renowned specialist in eating disorder treatment at the time, and just happened to be in our backyard. Dr. Larocca had convinced me that going into the hospital would help me. I wanted help. I was tired of throwing up, but I didn't seem to have a choice anymore. There were times when I didn't even have to try; the food would just start to come back up.

I didn't seem to be getting any thinner, and now everyone was watching my every move. I don't know that I was choosing treatment as much as I was running away from The Plan and the mess I'd made of my world.

Why did I have to say anything in front of Bobbie Nolan?! Mom might have just let that interaction go right on by, but I had to give it a witness. I hated myself.

For the first forty-eight hours of the program, patients couldn't have any contact with the outside world. Those were privileges you earned by eating your meals and following the rules of the program—and sometimes gaining weight.

I couldn't call or see my parents. Every morning the nurses passed along that Dad had called to check on me. I cried during every waking hour of those first two days—I was right back to being in first grade. The waking hours were endless.

The routine began very early as the doctor did his rounds between 4:00 a.m. and 6:00 a.m. The nurses would wake us up for weights and vitals before he arrived. We were required to go to the bathroom before heading down the hallway to be weighed, and we could wear only a hospital gown—no undergarments. That rule was to prevent us from putting rocks, or other items, in our underpants that would make it appear we weighed more than we did.

On that first morning, I was exhausted and petrified. I had that wave of nausea that I always get when I'm startled awake from a deep sleep. I waited for my roommate to use the bathroom and head down the hall. I was alone in the dark room when the tears started flowing again. I was now awake enough to be scared. As I walked down the hallway, I knew I'd made a horrible mistake. I had no business being here. The girls were all so skinny. Some were pushing poles on wheels that held bags of liquid food that flowed through the tube in their nose down to their stomach.

It was quickly evident that most of the girls had been here a while and there was a system. For most, the goal was to get in, get out, and get back to bed for a few precious moments of sleep before the doctor arrived. A few had actually showered and were wearing full face makeup. I stood toward the back of the line, silently crying, waiting until I was the last one in the hall.

I smiled at the kind nurse who tried to reassure me that I was going to be okay. She then gave me the lay of the land.

"Sit here and I'll do blood pressure and temp at the same time. Stand up, turn around, and step on the scale backward with your gown open in the back."

We weren't allowed to see our weight. I felt obese. I was certain the lady was wondering why in the world I was in the hospital. I knew what I weighed, and I was big. These girls were way better than me. I was a complete loser. A big, fat, loser who craved attention so much that she'd conned someone into thinking she needed to be in the hospital. I was mortified.

I went back to my bedroom and lay awake, crying, until word made it down the hall that the doctor had arrived. Everyone rushed into the dining room, in which there was an office the size of a broom closet. Breakfast would be at 7:00 a.m., followed by a full day of group and individual therapy. All of the girls who weren't showered and in full face makeup were hoping to be called first, so they could get a little more sleep before getting ready for the day.

I sat there crying quietly and looked around the room. There was a darling girl with one of those Madonna-like headbands with a big bow on top. She looked about my age. There were girls that were so skinny, I couldn't tell if they were women or girls. Their faces were so sunken they appeared wrinkly, but their bodies looked like pre-pubescent boys. There were older women—in their thirties—and some were even mothers.

I was the last one to be called. The newest patient was always last to be called. I walked into the tiny office, and Dr. Larocca closed the door. I could do nothing but cry. I couldn't say anything. He asked me why I was crying, and I just looked at him and cried some more.

"I won't hurt you," he said.

I nodded as I cried harder. I couldn't speak.

After a long silence, he said, "I'll see you tomorrow."

I went back down the hallway to my room. It was the last one on the right. I was glad for the long walk. I needed the exercise.

"Has anyone noticed anything about Missy?" said the nurse who was facilitating group therapy.

It was my third day, and it was the first group session of the morning. I was wearing my mint-green sweatpants and a black sweatshirt. Sitting on the couch next to one of the girls with a pole holding her bag of food, I was silently crying off the makeup I'd just applied.

"She always smiles. Even when she's crying," said the nurse, following a pregnant pause, to a group of blank-faced women.

This was a Kelley Girl thing. No matter what happened, especially when things seemed really bad, Mom's mantra was: "Just put a smile on your face and keep going." The nurse's comment made me smile even more. I was proud of myself for keeping a happy face through it all. I thought she was paying me a compliment.

This was the beginning of my self-esteem training. It was the first of many times throughout the years that I'd be told to accept myself exactly as I am in the moment. That's not what it sounded like on that day, though.

At best, it sounded like, "It's okay to cry, and you don't have to smile for the rest of us when you're sad."

Actually, I think even that was lost on me. What I really heard was, "You're not supposed to smile when you cry. You're doing it wrong."

I was determined to get it right. I wasn't the thinnest girl there, but I was going to be the best patient ever. I listened, I learned, I tried hard. I stopped smiling when I cried.

I talked in group therapy, and I really liked it. It was liberating to speak my fears and shameful behaviors and have others validate my worth despite the behaviors. I felt accepted for the first time in a long time. I fit in. I felt at home. I was well-liked by the other patients and the staff. I even had a favorite nurse, Patty, with whom I really bonded.

As I imagine happens in all types of recovery, one risk you run in a group setting is learning tricks of the trade that you hadn't tried before. There were many unsanctioned conversations about binging and purging, about hiding food and sneaking in exercise. I even learned about sex from the girl with the Madonna-bow headband. I didn't mean to. I didn't even know we were talking about sex.

I was sitting on her bed one afternoon and we were talking. She lived in Saint Louis and went to one of the public schools in a wealthier part of town. She was a senior and she had a boyfriend. We were talking about our boyfriends, and I started to tell her about how I wouldn't let my boyfriend touch my stomach—with clothes on—but I got embarrassed and stopped. She got very excited about having this conversation and urged me on.

"What? Tell me! When he looks at you? When he goes down on you?" I had no earthly idea what she was talking about.

I remember feeling like time had stopped. This was one of those moments when everyone in the class knew the answer but me, or when I was laughing at a joke that I didn't understand at all. I was nervous again and tried to replay the last few lines in my head, so that I could piece together what she meant.

Eventually, she just looked really disappointed and said, "Oh. Yeah, I don't like it when he touches my stomach either."

The other girl that schooled me on sex was a fourteen-year-old freshman. She was dating a senior. The good news was that I was aware that we were talking about sex. The bad news was that I still didn't really know what she was talking about. I guess I understood, but I just couldn't fathom her situation.

She was telling me that she wasn't sure if she'd had sex yet or not. She told me of a night when she was at a party drinking with her eighteen-year-old boyfriend, and she passed out. When she woke up there was blood on the sheets. I was confused by the waking up part—was that the next day? Did she spend the night with him? She was a freshman. Did her mom let her stay out late enough to fall asleep and wake up again? She said she asked him if they'd had sex, but he didn't really answer her.

After twenty-eight days of treatment, it was time to go home. I'd been taught meal plans and assertiveness. I'd been through group therapy and individual therapy. I'd learned the tricks of the trade—good and bad—and, of course, the added bonus of sex education.

I was afraid to go home.

Recovered, or Recovery?

Journal Entry from 2008, Forty Years Old

I gave up sugar three weeks ago. Last night, I dreamed of cookie dough! It wasn't the delicious, cold, rich, textured cookie dough you just mixed, or that comes in the yellow, Toll House wrapper. This cookie dough was in clear plastic wrap, and it was in the back of my car. It had been sitting in the sun for hours. It looked terrible. In this sorry, sugar-starved state, however, it looked like a tall drink of cold water in the middle of a desert.

In this dream, I debated back and forth whether I should eat it or not. Just one little lick. I plucked one chocolate chip out of the mess and popped it in my mouth. It was four seconds of pure bliss. Then, the guilt began. Oh, so guilty. I'm off the wagon. I had made it so long. I'm on the slippery slope. All that for nothing!

I woke up in a panic! Did I really cheat? The dream haunted me throughout the day today. It would be so easy to just grab a bite. I'm thin. People think it's crazy to give up sweets . . .

Journal Entry from 2019, Fifty-One Years Old

My arm is draped around the toilet seat, my feet curled beneath my bottom. I feel small. I think about what there is to say about this; it definitely feels like part of the story.

The first time I threw up my feelings was thirty-five years ago. I've only done it a handful of times in the past ten years. Tonight was one of them.

"Physical Therapy is not going to work." I looked up at the young woman as a tornado of thoughts swirled through my mind: surgeons always want to operate, hammers think everything is a nail, physical therapists think physical therapy will make a difference. What is she talking about? She's a physical therapist—of course physical therapy will help Robbie.

Maybe I did this. I've defined him by his disabilities and his prematurity, and now I've manifested a real problem. Major surgery. Surgery for people who really have cerebral palsy; not the mild version we were blessed with. Robbie has the kind people don't notice. She recommends seeing a surgeon.

I miss my dad.

I throw up.

I've met dozens of people recovering, or recovered, from an eating disorder over the years. I've remained friends with several women with whom I was in treatment over thirty years ago. Many say you never really get over it. I've uttered those words myself, and I've given this much thought throughout the process of writing this book.

Perhaps the reason people say it never goes away can be attributed to one of the primary personality traits associated with eating disorders—perfectionism.

Can I really say I'm recovered when I'm not perfectly recovered? At times I still feel anxious about the size of my body, or the cellulite on my legs, or feel the crumbling thought that I'm not a good enough person because my body doesn't look like a twenty-five-year-old model. Or a forty-year-old model.

Can I say I'm recovered when just three years ago I made myself throw up in a moment of extreme discomfort and overwhelm? What about if sometimes I punish myself for eating too much by exercising extra hard?

Perhaps quibbling over semantics to describe the period of life after the initial onset of an eating disorder isn't important. Recovery is as personal and individual as the stories of each of our lives. I don't like to say I'm recovered. Keeping those unwanted thoughts at bay or listening to what they're really trying to tell me requires vigilance, and I'm still susceptible to that struggle. I never want to forget that.

I describe myself as "someone with a history of eating disorders." I've had periods of both bulimia and anorexia. While I haven't been in the throes of behaviors that require hospitalization in decades, evaluating my body, what I've eaten, what I haven't eaten, how my clothes fit, and whether or not I look fat, thin, athletic, or flabby still occurs regularly.

These thoughts are typically fleeting and pass through like the millions of other thoughts that I don't control. My days no longer center around dieting, measuring, comparing, binging, or purging.

And I never diet.

In times of extreme or prolonged stress, however, the thoughts become more pervasive, and the stressful situation is compounded by that fear I first remember experiencing when I was six years old. My reactions are rarely extreme, and the life I've built is more important to me than stepping into that dark world. But there are times I open the door and take a peek. This usually takes the form of temporarily restricting my eating or increasing my exercise.

How long I linger in the shadows depends on how quickly I remember to use these unsettling thoughts and feelings for good. These compulsions are usually the first sign that I'm not being true to myself, that I'm feeling out of control, or that I'm acting from a place of fear.

Some people give a name to their eating disorder as a way to dissociate, to remind them that those thoughts and compulsions are separate from who they are. It has a life of its own; it's an enemy or a trickster whom they recognize immediately and laugh at or scold, then turn away and change their thought or choose a different action.

I believe that having named the eating disorder would have been helpful to me in those early days. This wasn't a tool that was taught to me. The self-esteem training at the hospital and subsequent group therapy focused on changing thought patterns related to self-worth and the relative nature of body image. In response to a bad thought, I was taught to choose a good thought. The idea was to retrain my brain by building new neural pathways, or mental habits, so that over time my default thought patterns would be healthier ones.

This was easier said than done, and I didn't understand that the thoughts that cross our mind don't define us. My identity became intertwined with my eating disorder. I felt shame for not having high self-esteem, and the negative thoughts just kept coming.

Naming the eating disorder and considering the collection of associated thoughts as something separate from my true self may have helped me grasp the distinction between having a thought, choosing a thought, and attaching to a thought.

Considering how breathing works has helped me understand this concept. Breathing is an autonomic function. It happens without me thinking about it. However, I can turn my attention to my breathing and make a breath cycle longer or shorter, and I can even stop a cycle by holding my breath. My breath isn't me.

Thoughts happen. I don't know what my next thought is going to be. As with my breath, when I center my attention on my thoughts, I can create a new one, evaluate an old one, or even try to stop the next one from coming, which people sometimes achieve through transcendental meditation. My thoughts aren't me.

I now understand that the thoughts *we attach to* affect our energy, emotions, and actions. In the throes of an active eating disorder, I'm fully attached to thoughts that support a belief system that equates lovability to a thin and small body.

Learning to choose a thought that feels better and is aligned with the beautiful nature of our true selves—which is love—is a helpful skill for managing life. As Gary Zukav said in The *Seat of the Soul, "When we align our thoughts, emotions, and actions with the highest part of ourselves, we are filled with enthusiasm, purpose, and meaning. Life is rich and full."*

I have been asked countless times, "How did you get over it?" The question often comes from a place of desperation by the loved one of someone who suffers this plight. I have turned that question over in my mind for years, equally desperate for a profound answer that will help these people. Clearly, medical treatment and the support of the recovery community played a significant role. However, none of that would have made a real difference if I hadn't found reasons to step back into life.

The simplest answer to how I "got over" my eating disorder, multiple times, is that each time something caught my attention that was more enticing than the dark, empty pit of being sick. And, I couldn't have both. Eventually, that one enticing thing expanded my awareness or social circle and became more than one thing. Slowly, my life became full of people I connected with, goals I wanted to achieve, and opportunities I couldn't fully experience while binging, purging, dieting, or over-exercising.

Now, in my mind's eye, my eating disorder is a golden ball of thorns. It's easy to focus on the sparkly gold color and forget about the bloody pain caused by its prickly edges. This thorny golden ball now lives in a sphere of soft, beautiful, shimmery protective light reflecting pink, purple, and gold. There's a tiny fairy with iridescent blue wings, named Vigilance, who guards the ball, so I remember it's no longer an option.

The wayward thoughts are a glare coming from the protective light, like when the sun bounces off metal and momentarily blinds you. Or Vigilance emits a high-pitched noise by moving her wings quickly, grabbing my attention so that I know I'm off track, that I'm out of balance, that I'm getting caught up in the gold luster of thinness and control, forgetting about the thorns. It's never really about the food. It's never really about the weight, or the fat, or the muscle, or the size of my pants.

The gift of my eating disorder was that it catapulted me into a lifelong journey of self-discovery, existentialism, hard work, and resilience. The beautiful, brilliant light reminds me that instead of staying mired in the thoughts and behaviors of disordered eating, I used it as a springboard to launch me into a full life.

Part 2:
Underlying Issues . . . It's Never Really about the Food

Chapter 1
Trauma

Alayna

According to neuroscientist Dr. Jill Bolte Taylor, author of *Whole Brain Living*, the left and right parts of our brains each contain a "thinking" part and an "emotions" part. The left "emotions" part is what remembers past experiences. If you were bitten by a German Shepherd as a child, your left brain will freak out when you see a German Shepherd. It's there to protect you from getting hurt like you did in the past. It's what reminds you of your trauma.

There's an ongoing joke between some of my friends and me that sophomore year of high school was the worst year of our lives. Although we laugh about it, we're not lying. We were all going through a tough time as sophomores, but we all kept our struggles a secret until years later. There wasn't one singular cause of my anxiety and eating disorder, but a lot of it is rooted in trauma for me.

It's difficult for me to admit that I've experienced trauma. It's easier to laugh with my friends, in a self-deprecating way, about how I used to be anorexic. But there was real trauma in my past, and most of us, whether we acknowledge it or not, have experienced trauma as well.

Sophomore Dance was traumatizing. I type this slowly, because I never want anyone to believe that *they* traumatized me. That's a big reason why I kept it to myself for so long, because the last thing I wanted was for my friends to blame themselves for my struggles. I can feel the hesitation in my fingers to get these words out, because it still brings me pain to talk about.

I was going through a lot of self-discovery sophomore year, and I was trying my hardest to gain social status at my Catholic all-girls high school. My pursuit of happiness was about getting fake tans, getting invited to parties, getting perfect pictures to post, meeting boys, and making sure I was noticed. The way I saw it, Sophomore Dance was a perfect opportunity to gain some social points!

I got my fake tan, my short red dress, my nails done, my heels high, and my smile on. I was bursting with excitement as my friends and I drove to another girl's house to get pictures taken before the dance. There were some girls I hadn't met before, so I made sure to laugh at their jokes and tell them they looked pretty. There was also a kitchen counter filled with snacks: Chick-fil-A nuggets, veggies and hummus, tortilla chips and salsa, and more. I didn't have an eating disorder at the time, but I was definitely food conscious.

"Make sure you girls eat something before you go," said one of the moms.

"Yea, thanks, mom for making me look fat in my dress," said the daughter while rolling her eyes. I laughed with my friends at her comment. I had one Chick fil-A nugget. Another skinny girl had three carrots with no hummus. Noted.

The dance itself was pretty fun. I love dancing. But all of our minds were focused on what would happen after. The most important part of the night: the after-party. God, I wish I could slap my younger self across the face for thinking the after-party was more important. I should have enjoyed my time at the dance.

The last song played and that was our cue to put our heels back on and sprint to our designated cars. I was in a car with my grade-school friends, so I was comfortable. We blared music and began drinking vodka straight out of the bottle on our way to the after-party. I danced and sang with the windows down, knowing that this was about to be a night I would always remember.

We arrived at the house of the girl who was hosting the party, and my stomach did a flip. I didn't know why, but I was suddenly nervous. I took another shot to ease my nerves. As we walked in, girls and guys started filing in behind us. My friends and I changed into our party clothes in a bedroom. I changed in a corner so no one would see my stomach exposed. Another shot.

"Come on! Let's go downstairs and fuck shit up!" I heard a voice yell.

Sure, I guess so, I thought.

As I walked down to the unfinished basement, it seemed like the number of people there had quadrupled since I first arrived. *Be cool, be cool, be cool.* On my right was a game of beer pong, and behind it was a couch where a few couples were starting to make out. To my left it was too dark to see what people were doing, and in front of me more selfies and pictures were being taken. Rap music that I pretended to know the words to, colorful lights flashing and filling the room, guys, girls, handles of vodka, beer, seltzers. *Wait, where are my friends? I need my friends. Why am I not having fun?*

"Hey! Thank fucking goodness! I've been looking for you," I said to my friend as she stumbled toward me.

With barely audible speech she replied, "Who are you?" and was pulled the other direction to take more shots. My best friend just looked me in the eyes and asked who I was.

My eyes welled with tears as I started breathing heavily. I decided to go upstairs and calm down in the bathroom. I passed some more people making out on my way up. *Why don't any guys want to do that with me? I'm just not as hot as those girls.*

I stumbled a little bit into the bathroom, and sat on the toilet seat, sobbing into my hands. People knocked on the door to throw up, but I wasn't ready to be seen.

Finally, another knock came, and a familiar voice said, "I have to pee sooo bad."

It was one of my friends, so I opened the door and let her in. She saw my face and immediately gave me a hug.

I guess the mascara dripping down my fake-tanned face was enough for her to tell that I was upset. She asked me, "Did a boy do something to you?"

"What? No. I just . . . got a little overwhelmed," I replied.

"I get that way too sometimes. Why don't we go back downstairs together?" She made me feel safe as she helped me wipe my tears away and take some deep breaths.

We walked out of the bathroom and I saw two girls in the corner of the kitchen across the house. One of the girls was kneeling by the other one, who was sitting in a chair. I walked closer and quickly realized that the girl in the chair was my friend who asked who I was just 10 minutes ago. Before I knew it I was sprinting over to her.

"Oh my gosh, what in the hell happened?!" I asked, seeing a pool of vomit on the floor.

"She just had too much to drink," the girl replied calmly.

We took turns sticking our fingers down my best friend's throat in efforts to make her throw up: a technique I would try on myself a few months later when I thought I ate too much.

I began to sob once again, saying, "You're gonna be okay, Sweetie, I'm right here. I'm not leaving." She wasn't throwing up and she wasn't swallowing water. I tried to pry open her eyelids, only to reveal the whites of her eyes. My best friend began foaming at the mouth.

"Alayna! Your friend is calling for you in the bedroom," said a voice. I told my unconscious friend I would be right back, and I sprinted to the bedroom. I found my other friend on the floor, leaning her back against the bed, holding a cardboard box filled with puke.

"Alayna, please talk to my parents on the phone," she muttered with her eyes shut. I took a deep breath, tried my best to sober up, and picked up the phone.

"Hi, this is Alayna. She had too much to drink. I'm sorry, but can you please come get us?" I told her mom.

"Don't worry," I assured my friend after getting off the phone, "your dad is on the way to pick you up." She gave me a thumbs up as she shivered on the floor.

I told her I would be right back, and I rushed back into the kitchen, slipping on a pile of puke, only to find my other friend gone. *She couldn't have gone far.* I checked the bathroom, but in the bathtub I saw a big guy throwing up on himself while his friends laughed at him. Frantically, I kept searching until I found my friend in another bedroom, lying limply on the bed. I knelt beside her and brushed her hair back with my fingers, which were still covered in mucus from the back of her throat.

I heard a man's voice yell, "Whose dad is outside in a van?!"

"I think that's my friend's dad!" I said. I ran back over to the conscious friend, scooped my hands under her arms to help her up, and walked her outside to her dad's car. I helped her into the passenger seat, and told her dad that he should take my other friend, too, because she was unconscious and foaming at the mouth. At that point, I turned around to see my best friend being carried like a cradled child to the car by the host's dad.

I watched her being placed into the backseat of the van, and the next thing I knew, the van was gone. My vision was hazy, and I was feeling the spins start to kick in.

I went back inside to pack up my things and make sure I had everything with me. At least I still had my other friends and a sleepover at another girl's house to look forward to. I found my small Lululemon bag in the bedroom next to my friend's puke-filled cardboard box. I grabbed it and headed back out to find my other friends so I could get the hell out. But suddenly, the house was empty and quiet. My friends were gone. The host parents saw me standing by the front door and asked, "Do you need us to give you a ride home?"

"No, I'm good. I'll call my parents," I said.

I looked at my phone for the first time all night. It was almost 2:00 a.m. I dialed my mom's number. *Please pick up.*

"Hi, mom. I'm sorry. Can you please come get me?" I said with a shaky voice.

"What the hell happened? Yes, we'll come get you," my mom said.

"Thanks for having me," I told the parents, and I stumbled out of that front door. Seeing my parents' car in front of the house gave me the biggest sense of relief.

They watched me walk to the car, my shirt covered in brown puke stains and mascara marks. I plopped into the back seat and began, once again, to sob. Only this time, I couldn't breathe.

My parents told me I was in big trouble for being irresponsible. This only made me cry harder. I couldn't stop crying enough to tell them what happened.

I cried myself to sleep that night. When I woke up, I looked at snapchat and saw that all of my friends had a big sleepover and went to breakfast together. My two best friends ended up getting home ok, but my unconscious friend had gone to the hospital for alcohol poisoning. She recovered and went home later that day. Two other boys from that party also went to the hospital.

I explained to my parents everything that went down at the party, but I thought I was being way too sensitive about it. My brother told me, "Yea, that's shitty, but everyone has to take their turn being the responsible one at a party." *This happens all the time. You're not that special,* I told myself.

These were my thoughts, and sometimes they still are. But the way that this event affected me was profound. I slowly started isolating myself after that night, and, with a combination of many other factors, I developed an eating disorder. This event in no way was the singular cause of my eating disorder, because I was already an anxiety-ridden teenager. However, it was a night that caused me nightmares for months. One night, I dreamt that my friends locked me in a closet and never came back to get me.

Another night, I dreamt that I was crying in front of my friends, who were all facing me and looking into my eyes with straight faces, and they turned around and left one by one. I believe it was the feeling of unintentional abandonment and loneliness that traumatized me.

I still cry sometimes when I am out with friends at a party. I now have what I call an "anxiety shiver," where my upper body flinches and I make a shivering noise with my mouth. It started a month or so after Sophomore Dance, and I didn't know until a couple years later that many people with anxiety develop nervous "tics" like my shivers.

Trauma is very real and very individual. It's a beautiful thing that our brains remember the details surrounding the trauma. If we're bit by a certain kind of dog, our brains want us to remember. Holding onto details like that helps us avoid being retraumatized—at least by another German Shepherd.

Getting help with processing the effects of trauma can make a big difference in your ability to move forward in a healthy way. I eventually addressed the emotional effects of the Sophomore Dance with my therapist, and it was critical to my recovery.

Trauma

Melissa

"Missy, you are a tough cookie. You are going to be okay. Just try to stay calm." This was Colleen, my eldest sister, when it was her turn to say goodbye before they took me to surgery.

They were all lined up to take their turn at my bed. I felt like I was at my own wake. People filled the room, keeping their distance from my bed unless I started to cry or needed something. There were hushed, tearful conversations, and lots of hugging.

The day had started early with a splitting headache that woke me up at 6:00 a.m. When we arrived at the maternity ward, I announced, "I'm 26 weeks pregnant, I have a headache, and my doctor told me to come here."

My memory of that first hospital is beige. The room was nondescript, the people who worked with me had little to say, and it was very quiet like we were the only ones there. They had placed a catheter in me so I wouldn't have to get out of bed, and every so often someone came in to ask me a question.

Then came this pronouncement from a man in a lab coat whose role wasn't clear to me: "You aren't 26 weeks pregnant."

"What? Yes I am." Complete confusion.

"No, based on the first day of your last period, you are 25 weeks, 5 days pregnant," he said with a seriousness that seemed ridiculous to me.

"I was rounding up." Likely accompanied by an eyeroll.

"Well at this stage of the game, every day counts."

What game? I'm not here to have a baby. I'm here to get rid of my headache.

The previous day, I'd had an appointment with my obstetrician. Two weeks previous to that visit, I had met this doctor for the first time in my pregnancy. The pregnancy had been rough on my body and when I would share my symptoms and concerns with my regular obstetrician I was left feeling unheard, dismissed, and dramatic. After a particularly frustrating appointment with him, I called the doctor my sisters used and asked if he would see me.

Dr. Colton saw me the very next day and listened closely as I shared the history of my pregnancy, including an anomaly on my 20-week ultrasound, and persistent nausea. He said he was happy to work with me, took my vitals, conducted an in-office ultrasound just to make sure I was stable, and asked that I return two weeks later.

At that next visit, I said, "I just don't feel the baby moving as much."

"Let's just do a quick ultrasound for peace of mind," Dr. Colton said as he rolled a machine next to the examination table.

After moving the wand through the cold gel across my whale belly for what seemed like forever, he said, "Have you been leaking fluid?"

"No. Uh, I don't think so."

"Are you sure? No wetness in your underpants that you have noticed?"

"Well, sometimes when I go to the bathroom I notice that I didn't quite make it in time because there are a few drops in my underwear," I said sheepishly.

"That wasn't urine, it was amniotic fluid."

I looked at him confused and embarrassed. He explained that there was only a golf ball-sized amount of amniotic fluid left in the amniotic sac. I would later learn that there were blood clots in the placenta and a slow leak, which is why the wetness I noticed wasn't alarming to me. I thought it was urinary incontinence, which is not even one of the weirder things that happens to your body when you're pregnant. Like dark spots on your skin, and increased hair growth.

"We are going to draw some blood and then you need to go home. Your blood pressure is high, so for the rest of the pregnancy, you will be at home resting. I will call you later with the lab results."

I was already scheduled for a Level II ultrasound at the hospital the next day, so when the lab results indicated markers for preeclampsia, a dangerous blood pressure condition in pregnancy that can cause seizure, stroke, and even death of the mother, we agreed that I could stay home until that appointment. He suggested I be packed and ready to stay in the hospital until the baby was born and gave the caveat that if I got a headache or started feeling worse, I was to call him immediately.

After correcting my math on the pregnancy, no one had come into my room for a while. I knew John, my then husband, was around somewhere but he must have been getting coffee when I felt a rush of warm fluid, that I could not control, pour out of me.

I pressed the call button, and spoke to the staticky, too-loud voice coming out of the holes on the remote control. "I wet my bed. I think the catheter came out."

"Your catheter is fine," the nurse told me, eying me oddly. Presumably this was the golf ball-sized amount of fluid that had been noted on the ultrasound the day before, but no one ever acknowledged the matter. There were bigger fish to fry. The hospital I was in didn't have a Level III Neonatal Intensive Care Unit (NICU) so they couldn't handle a baby of this gestation. I started to feel worse as the minutes passed, and the decision was made to transfer me by ambulance to a nearby hospital that was equipped to manage our care.

At the next hospital, I was in a large room and there was lots of activity. My arms were anchored to the bed by an IV and a blood pressure cuff. There were electric wires dripping from foamy stickers on my belly, flowing to the machine tracking our heart rates and other vital signs. Magnesium sulfate, "mag," was running through my veins to lower my blood pressure. This was the best drug at the time for the situation, and one that was known to make you feel terrible. It was living up to its reputation.

When I closed my eyes, I saw dinosaurs lining up to race. When I opened my eyes, I was back at my wake. People were grouped at what felt like the bottom of the room, *Am I on a hill?*, and new visitors kept arriving. When the sadness of my family became too much, I would close my eyes and watch the dinosaurs.

Three of my sisters, my brother, my aunt, John's parents, and even the pastor from our church were there. This was January 2002. Texting was not a function available on all phones and there was no social media. As the family members piled up, especially those who were school teachers, I started to understand the magnitude of the situation. They had each been phoned and told the situation was precarious.

"Meghan is coming home," Dad said with a smile. I looked at him and tried to calculate the meaning of my youngest sister, who was in law school in Denver, coming home at the end of January.

John started rubbing my feet. *Oh, God. I'm in trouble. Meghan is coming home and John hates feet.*

The doctor and nurse stood together next to the window. Dad leaned against a counter at the bottom of the room, his arms crossed, resting on his big belly. John stood at the foot of my bed. It was just the five of us now and there were decisions to be made.

It had been so long since the baby had moved, that I no longer felt connected to it. The doctor shared the mortality rate for babies at this level of gestation. I don't remember the number, just the anger of my husband at the doctor's negativity.

The nurse responded to John's outburst with a compassionate look and asked, "Do you want the baby baptized?"

My big, strong father who could fix anything, had transformed into a sad little boy. I locked eyes with him, seeking an answer. Not just to that question but to everything that was happening. I couldn't grasp it. He gave me a helpless nod, then his chin dropped to his chest.

The surgery was white. The room was white, the specialist delivering the baby had white hair, and a white sheet blocked my view. The nurse sitting next to me held a cold, white washcloth on my forehead as I threw-up in the emesis tray.

From behind the white sheet, I heard the pretty blonde nurse with big, blue eyes who would baptize the baby say, "It's a girl!"

What? I was confused. Although we had chosen not to find out the sex of the baby at our 20-week ultrasound, I was certain it was a boy.

Seconds later, my husband corrected her with pride. "It's a BOY!"

The nurse was now at my bedside holding the baby in her two hands. He was so tiny, weighing in at one pound, five ounces. What happened next will be one of the moments that play back to me when I'm seeing the highlight reel of my life, right before I pass on to the next realm. The tiny baby we called Robbie opened one eye—a wink—and spoke to my soul: "It's okay, Mama."

I tried so hard to hold it in so that Robbie's soul's first memory of me would be as beautiful as mine was of him, but I couldn't control it. I turned my head and threw up.

My struggle with anorexia began shortly thereafter. I had gained 40 pounds during that first pregnancy. The baby weighed one. He was in the NICU for 113 days, on a ventilator for nine weeks, and oxygen for nine months. The medical team told me the best thing I could do for the baby while he was in the hospital was pump breast milk. It was recommended that I stop taking the antidepressant I had been on, in some form, since I was 18 years old, because there could be traces of it in the breast milk.

This did not go well.

I became very depressed. In addition to still being very sick from the preeclampsia, my baby was in the hospital on a ventilator and we didn't know what his long-term prognosis was, or if he would even survive. Much of my 40-pound weight gain was fluid due to high blood pressure, and pumping breast milk burned a lot of calories. The weight began to fall off fast.

Over the four months in the NICU, I would often skip meals to be with the baby, or meet with a doctor. I remember my friend, Tina, bringing me St. Louis Bread Company for lunch one day, and right as we were heading to the parents' break room to eat I was offered the opportunity to "Kangaroo" with Robbie. This is when the baby, who is only wearing a diaper, is placed on the parent's chest. It's skin-on-skin contact and helps with bonding, which is important for every baby and difficult to achieve when the baby can only be held once a day, and that is if everything is going well.

I never passed up a chance to Kangaroo with Robbie, so my stomach growled and ached with hunger as Tina sat with Robbie and me through lunch, which would have been my first meal that day. Yes, I was skipping that meal to Kangaroo with the baby, not to lose weight. But, what happened to breakfast?

The old thought patterns were activated the minute people started commenting on how fast I was losing the baby weight, and situations like Kangarooing through lunch felt good. It would perpetuate weight loss. I felt disciplined and in control of *something*.

Eventually, I was allowed to take the antidepressant again, which helped with the crying and depression, but the die was cast on the weight loss. I convinced myself and others that I wasn't trying to lose weight. That was only half true. The bigger problem was that I had a huge aversion to gaining weight so as I lost it, I did whatever it took to keep it off.

Eight months after the birth of Robbie, who we now call Robin (she/her), I was pregnant again. Because of the course of my first pregnancy, I was under the care of a specialist who ordered bed rest after about 20 weeks. I did have preeclampsia again, but it was not severe, and I was under careful watch.

Bed rest was tough for my eating disorder brain. All I did was lay in bed, eat, watch Netflix DVDs (it was 2003), and buy things on eBay that we would need to manage two babies who couldn't walk. Since a dramatic increase in water weight could be an indicator of the worsening of preeclampsia, I had to weigh myself every day and report it to the hospital.

This did not go well.

After about four weeks of bed rest and watching my weight rise, I decided to go on a diet. I started skipping lunch and stopped snacking. I began to keep careful watch over what went into my mouth. No one noticed and it is unlikely there was any effect on the baby. Erin was born five weeks early, and spent only five days in the NICU. The dieting during that pregnancy had once again activated the thought patterns that would drive my anorexic tendencies for a few years to come.

With two babies fourteen months apart it was easy to be too busy to eat. I had gotten a trainer that I could see early in the morning before the babies woke up. The weight was off but my shape had changed a little and I was determined to lose what I thought was a pooch in my stomach. I asked the 22-year-old trainer who'd never had a baby, "Is it possible for my body to go back to the way it was before my pregnancies?"

She replied, "Yes, it just depends on how hard you work."

Challenge accepted.

"How much weight have you lost?!" I had just walked into my boss's office. The babies were in daycare and Erin, the youngest, was a little over a year old. "I can see your rib cage."

I was stunned. *Are you supposed to answer when your boss asks you how much weight you've lost?* I dismissed the comments with a laugh and assured him I never miss a meal or a snack. Inside, I was so proud of myself. I had never been so thin.

About a week after Erin turned two, my life took an unexpected turn. It was actually more like I turned a corner and ran straight into an oncoming train. I needed to get divorced. I had two kids, one with special needs. Four months earlier, I had stopped working because Robin had been diagnosed with autism, and adding 20 hours a week of therapy to the six we already had going was just too much for me. I needed a break.

I didn't try to lose weight. It just happened. And while I really believed that, I now understand that my eating disorder brain kicks in the minute something traumatic happens. And, this was definitely trauma. In less than three years, I had two premature babies and multiple diagnoses that classified Robin as special needs. Now, I was facing a divorce that I didn't see coming.

It was Erin's therapist, Julie, who confronted me about my weight and need for treatment. Erin was still really young so the therapy for her consisted of drawing pictures and learning to identify feelings. The therapist and I spent most of the time talking about my issues with raising the kids by myself. I didn't have time for my own therapist. If I was texting you right now, I would insert the eye-roll emoji at my own ridiculousness. The three-year-old had a therapist but the needs of the heartbroken, anorexic mother of two toddlers—one with special needs—who worked full time, did not rise to the level of therapy-worthy.

"I think you need to see my friend Kim McCallum. She has an eating disorder clinic here in town and I can call her for you and see if she has time to talk to you," Julie said.

"I'm not trying to lose weight," I responded.

"I know. You've said that. I just think she can help you make sure you don't continue down a path that leads to not being able to take care of your kids."

Gulp. An image of the pregnant lady who was in eating disorder treatment with me appeared in my mind. "I don't want to be a mom and still be dealing with this." That is what I had told myself and my therapist.

How in the world did I get here?

Many people can trace the beginning of their eating disorder behaviors to the period following a traumatic event. For me, this is true with the onset of anorexia in my thirties but not necessarily with the onset of bulimia in my teens. Of course, sometimes people can't access the memories of a traumatic event, so that doesn't necessarily mean I didn't experience trauma before I became bulimic.

There have been many studies on the prevalence of trauma in eating disorder patients. The consensus seems to be that people with eating disorders are more likely to have experienced a traumatic event than people without eating disorders. The blog post "The Relationship Between Trauma and Eating Disorders" on the Center for Discovery website, says this connection is because many behaviors associated with eating disorders are also used as coping mechanisms in response to trauma. "An individual may feel out of control or powerless after experiencing a traumatic event and as a result, they use restricting or binging behaviors to control that aspect of their life in order to hide their feelings of shame, hopelessness, and fear."

The title for this section of the book states that it's never really about the food. Eating disorder behaviors often begin as a maladaptive response to life issues, such as trauma, or belief systems shaped by diet culture, such as perfectionism. In the following chapters, we will continue to share stories that exemplify how specific life issues and beliefs fed our eating disorders and how we now manage those to remain free of the disease and fully live.

Chapter 2
Fear of Growing Up

Alayna

My sixteenth birthday is the day I remember as my deepest depressive state. I didn't want to grow up. Sixteen came with responsibilities I didn't think I was ready for. At the time, I wasn't aware that I didn't want to grow up. In fact, I wasn't self-aware at all. I just thought I was anxious and depressed for no reason.

On the day of my birthday, I went to take my driving test. It's safe for you to assume that I was already in a sad mood all day, and the test was making me anxious. But I'd been reading a manual for new drivers—like a perfectionist would—so I figured I had it in the bag. My assigned cop was a woman who looked to be about six feet tall and had her wiry hair in a low, tight bun.

As soon as I got in the car with the lady cop, she barked, "Brights . . . turn them on!" *Holy shit. I'm gonna fail. This lady thinks I'm stupid. Why did no one tell me where my brights are?!*

I just shrugged my shoulders and she scribbled on a piece of paper. The rest of the test felt like a failure to me because it started out on a bad note. I hit the curb when I parallel parked. Today that's something I'd laugh at myself for, but my sixteen-year-old anxiety-ball viewed it as a failure.

I passed the test with an 82 percent. I broke down in tears once I was out of the car.

The lady cop was taken aback by my crying and said, "Honey, you know you passed, right?"

I nodded my head yes and climbed back into the passenger's seat to go home with my mom. I really didn't know why I was so upset, but it makes sense to me now. I'd just been given the responsibility of driving for the rest of my life, and it was freaking me out. I couldn't even imagine how I was going to get through the rest of the day, let alone the rest of my life. It was overwhelming to grow up.

The only thing I focused on was the weight listed on my driver's license. That gave my mind something to grab on to. I came home from the driving test and climbed the stairs straight up to my room to nap. *Maybe if I sleep hard enough I could sleep straight through this horrible day.*

My brother came home from college to surprise me that night, and I heard him walk into the house and yell, "Helloooo!" I pretended to be asleep, but I felt a smile start to form on my face. I heard my mom whispering to him downstairs. I kept hearing her whisper the word "she" and that was enough to know it was about me. I was humiliated and felt like a problem in the family.

Next, I heard Nathan's ankles cracking as he walked up the stairs and heard him open my door slowly. I pretended to wake up slowly. I didn't think I had a smile left in me, but I looked up at Nathan and couldn't help but show my teeth. I jumped up and gave him a big hug. At that moment I felt like my real self again, so I held on tight. It's important to hold on to those around you that know who you truly are so that when you're lost, they're there to remind you what it feels like to be found.

Two of my best friends came to take me out to dinner that night as a surprise. Little did they know I wanted nothing to do with celebrating my birthday, let alone going out to eat Mexican food . . . which was on the avoid-at-all-costs food list. I knew I should be grateful for what they were doing for me, so I dug as deep as I could to maintain my smile. The smile was more painful than my actual feelings because it was incredibly fake.

That night after getting Mexican food, my best friend (since kindergarten) sat in my basement with me as I scrolled through my phone. She suggested we get ice cream, and that's when I couldn't do it anymore.

"Oh wow, my stomach *really* hurts. I think I need to go to bed soon. Sorry," I said with tears forming.

How was I supposed to explain to my best friend that even she couldn't pull me out of my thoughts? There's nothing more heartbreaking than shutting out someone you love. I was aware that I was pushing her away, and it hurt like hell, but I thought it was my only option. Even if I wanted to tell her how I was feeling inside, she wouldn't understand, and I didn't want anyone to help me. *This is something I need to deal with on my own. Don't be a bitch, Alayna. Don't be a burden.*

Eventually, my friend left. My parents didn't want her to go. I could tell. They liked seeing me smile, and they knew that as soon as she left, the smile would leave too. They did everything in their power to keep that fake smile on my face for the rest of the night. Presents! That should do it! I got tickets to see my favorite sports team . . . the Saint Louis Blues hockey team. God, it broke my heart to be an ungrateful bitch, so I prayed that they wouldn't see through my fake smile. I opened the rest of my presents, sitting on a stool and bouncing my left leg up and down. *Keep going, keep going, just a little longer.* I don't really remember the rest of that night. I'm not sure if I talked to my parents or if I texted my friend. All I remember is the shame and guilt I felt for eating Mexican food as I cried myself to sleep.

I missed a lot in my seventeenth year of life.

Another part of growing up was going through puberty. I still hate that word. It kinda makes me cringe. I was a super late bloomer, since blooming late runs in the family, and I was also very active, which can slow down the process. Once I turned sixteen and still hadn't gotten my period, it was standard protocol for my pediatrician to make sure everything was functioning properly inside my body. I figured not getting my period was the luckiest thing to ever happen to me—my friends made periods sound like death. On the contrary, not getting your period can be extremely dangerous down the road and can cause major problems with fertility and a bunch of other issues I blocked out of my mind. The main reason I didn't want my period was because I thought it meant I'd gain weight and have a woman's body. Based on my growth charts, I was probably just about to get my period, and then I dropped weight dramatically. Significant weight loss postpones periods, which is why many women with anorexia lose their periods.

My dietitian was the first person to tell me that I needed to get my period. She said, "Your period is a beautiful sign of womanhood. You're no longer a little girl, and you must stop trying to keep your little girl body." Her words struck home. It clicked in my head at that moment. I was physically trying to stay a little girl, so I wouldn't have to face the responsibilities and fears that come with being an adult.

From that point on, getting my period became a major symbolic event. It would mean that there was no going back to being a little girl. That's why it was so scary. And that's why my mom threw a little party for me when it finally came—a few weeks after I turned seventeen.

Not only that, but it was also just a couple of weeks after I hit the weight goal my dietitian had set for me. It all aligned perfectly. When I got my period, my face felt like it was on fire. My heart pounded out of my chest. But I smiled because I felt like I was no longer a slave to my eating disorder.

I'm eighteen right now as I write this. I'm an adult. I've been getting my period for over a year now. I'm a woman, as weird as it is to say that, and I love it for the most part. I grew up, and I continue to get new responsibilities piled high on my plate. For example, as I write, I'm seven days away from moving away from home and into my college dorm. How's that for growing up? Of course, I'm scared, anxious, nervous, hesitant, and sad.

So, how am I dealing with it? I tell myself: *You know what it's like to postpone your life, and you didn't gain anything from doing so. So shed a few tears and move forward. The next phase of life is one you don't want to miss.*

Growing up is an opportunity, not a responsibility.

Fear of Growing Up

Melissa

What's in a Name?

In my first-grade class, there were two girls named Melissa. These days, teachers solve the confusion by adding the first initial of the student's last name. If that were my experience, I would have been Melissa K., and the other girl would have been Melissa H. I guess that was too many syllables, so Mrs. Hellweg said one of us had to be called Missy. She put the two of us in a corner and said that we had to work it out; there could be only one Melissa.

Two thoughts on this: 1) We didn't have work-it-out skills at age six, on day one of first grade, and 2) This wasn't a small decision. These would be our names for the rest of grade school, and in my case, because I went to high school with the same kids, it would be until I graduated.

This is how I remember the conversation going:

"I want to be Melissa," said Melissa H.

"Okay," I said dejectedly.

It didn't occur to me that I could push back and say I wanted to keep my name. My family called me Missy, but that felt like a special family nickname. I was Missy Mouse. Sometimes just Mouse. I didn't know any of the kids in that classroom, and I didn't want them calling me my special name.

This first taste of the real world taught me that it would steamroll me. I cried every morning on the way to school for the entire year. I missed my mom, and the environment felt cold and scary.

Fast Food

"Don't you want to play at recess with the other kids?" Mom asked. "You need to eat a little faster so you can go out and play."

There was a lot stress around lunch in first grade. Lunch was followed by recess. As soon as you finished eating, you could leave the table and head to the parking lot to play. I was a really slow eater. I took the entire lunch-recess break to eat and, of course, by the end of it, I was alone at a big table in the cafeteria. The teacher had reached out to my mom to rectify the situation.

I knew we were being watched. The lunch ladies (volunteer parents) walked around to supervise us. And then there were the nuns. The school principal was a nun. Her name was Sister Bernice, and she carried a pen and paper everywhere. She'd look at a table of kids, then bend her head and start writing something. For all we knew, she was making a grocery list for the convent, but the exercise was clearly designed to make us think she was taking notes on our behavior. She was like a somber, black-clothed Santa Claus from whom your best gift was a meeting with your parents. Or, staying in for recess.

I was nervous about the watchers. Especially the nuns. Sister Daneal also walked around. She made quirky comments, and you never knew if she was going to be silly—or mean. My mom was active as a room mother and Girl Scout leader over the years, but I wanted her to come to school at lunch. Maybe then I could have recess with her.

I tried to connect the words or behaviors that caused Sister Bernice's head to drop and the pen to move. I tried to eat faster. I didn't want my name on the list. Eventually, I learned to quicken my pace and join the kids on the parking lot for dodgeball.

Who Am I?

I used to recoil from the word *responsibility*. I was once involved in a community service project to help spruce up a middle school in my employer's neighborhood. As we entered the building, we were greeted with a huge billboard that said in letters that seemed to yell, "YOU ARE RESPONSIBLE FOR YOU." I immediately felt sick to my stomach. I was in my mid-thirties at the time, a single mother with a great career and two children. I was a responsible adult, and yet I felt small and scared when I saw that billboard.

In my experience, the word *responsibility* is often used as a weapon or a threat, instead of a tool of empowerment. When kids don't do their chores, we tell them they're irresponsible. We tell teens they need a job because they'll be responsible for paying their car insurance or college tuition. Responsibility is taught by default. It's taught as an appendage to all the things we must do to get through life. It's also used to assign blame. "It was your responsibility to get that done," or my favorite, "You can't control what others do to you, but how you respond is YOUR responsibility."

If I could rewrite the curriculum of growing up, one thing I'd start with is a celebration of all of the responsibilities kids have earned and will now take on as part of moving to the next grade. At each grade, those would change and become more important. Responsibility is serious, but it can be empowering if we introduce it correctly.

The belief that I needed to be chosen by a man for marriage was as much about my fear of responsibility as it was my search for an identity. Like most teenagers, I began to pull away from my family in my high school years. I didn't feel like I belonged. I was different—of course, we were all different—but my difference didn't make me special. I recall a trip to the eye doctor.

"Oh, you're a Kelley Girl! Are you the oldest, the cheerleader?" he asked.

"No, I'm third."

"Are you the singer? The athlete?" he asked.

"No."

"Well what are you famous for?" he prodded again.

Silence.

"Famous for being infamous?"

Pretty much.

I was an athlete. A good one. Not a great one. Not the one he was talking about. And I was a terrible singer. I was "a Kelley Girl." That was about as far as I got in terms of an identity. On several occasions, Dad asked me, "Why do you always take the hard road? You have two sisters who have paved the way, just follow them."

Dad was an only child, and I think he often, as a young boy, felt alone and scared while growing up. He had to forge his own way without the guidance or path of an older sibling to follow. He couldn't understand why I didn't take advantage of this luxury.

The thing is, their paths didn't work for me. My eldest sister and I had nothing at all in common at the time. I was close to my sister who's eighteen months older than me, and we did the same things throughout high school. When we were little, we put on performances for family and neighbors; she was the star, I was the director. That's only cute until you're about ten; after that it's just embarrassing. She went on to star in high school plays and sing in talent shows. We both played sports. I was good; she was great.

Many people tried to help me find my thing.

"It's okay, Missy, just sing us a song. It's just us!"

My parents and other relatives, perhaps my aunt or grandparents, sat on the plaid couch with encouraging eyes. I stood in front of the TV and reluctantly sang the song. Their faces said it all. They were very polite, but I felt ashamed.

"Draw what you see," Dad said as he placed the cereal box depicting a cartoon tiger in front of me, nudging the pencil and paper in my direction.

I could draw about as well as I could sing.

But I was good at school. I wasn't a straight-A student, which I really wanted to be, but I liked school, and I did well. When I started working at my dad's office, I got high praise for being his best worker. This was the kind of feedback I'd get for years to come, and it felt good. But I didn't trust myself to be in charge of myself, to create a life that would be worthy of the local ophthalmologist knowing who I am.

I grew up in an era where the social construct for women was changing. I witnessed a world where women were subordinate to men in the home and in their careers, if they even had a job outside of the home. This was reinforced in TV shows, commercials, movies, and the church. I was in the first generation of college graduates in my family, as were many of my friends.

Women were encouraged to get educated and plan careers, while at the same time, they were being bombarded with messages that the value of our bodies was determined by men and that getting married was still priority number one—a given for any real woman. The careers that most often depicted women were in caretaking fields, like teaching or nursing, or those supporting male executives.

"Just take shorthand as a backup," my father pleaded in my high school years.

Soon after, I started to stand out for something: the way I looked. One summer day after I'd graduated high school, Mom called me from her office and asked me to bring her something she'd left at home.

As I was getting ready to leave, she called again and said, "Make sure you look nice. I told them you're my pretty one."

That felt fantastic, yet it fed my belief that my worth was in my appearance.

"I don't want to have a mom's body," I'd say when someone asked what my end goal was with all my dieting.

My poor mother. I'd said that right to her beautiful face. A mom's body, not a *woman's* body, but a *mom's* body. In my mind, moms were women whose bodies were used for things like making and feeding babies. To me, they were rounder, bigger, and took up more space. They were noticed. They were used for other people.

In college, I started to gain confidence and build a sense of self that wasn't predicated on what my sisters did. I made good friends and spread my wings by joining a sorority in my junior year. This started off great because I met so many people. I didn't get into the sorority I wanted, so I settled for the one a few of my close friends had joined.

Early in pledge season, there was a fundraiser—a pledge auction. All the fraternities were invited, and one by one, the pledges were presented and auctioned off for a night. There were rules around what we could and couldn't be used for; it was all about selling the beauty of each girl and raising money for the next date party, of course.

I wore a form-fitting black outfit, one of my favorites for parties. As the stout, blond auctioneer with a pixie haircut spun me around, she pointed out, "That beautiful butt, gentlemen!" I was purchased by two guys for $50, the highest ransom yet. I didn't stick around for the rest of the auction. I ran home to binge and purge.

In hindsight, my eating disorder behavior was rebellion against all of it. I'm strong-willed. I didn't want a life that was determined by a man, and I wasn't suited to the caretaking careers. In what felt like a dangerous, scripted life with few opportunities for improvisation, my eating disorder allowed me to exit stage left. It was the doorway through which I could step out of a life that felt unsafe, out of control, and dedicated to chasing the moving target that is "enough."

Home Sweet Home

For years, I've used the word *home* to describe the feeling I get when I close my eyes and take a breath. I instantly feel grounded, secure, and content. I've also said, "It feels like home," when describing a romantic relationship that feels secure. Alternatively, when a person I was getting to know didn't feel right to me or left me feeling insecure, I'd describe the feeling as *homesick*.

In her book *Welcome Home*, author Najwa Zebian compares being anchored in who you are to being your own home. Alternatively, she notes that when you seek your identity in others or define yourself based on their acceptance or opinion of you, you're emotionally homeless.

I spent most of my life building homes in other people or searching for someone who found my room worthy of their home. I searched for that feeling of groundedness, acceptance, and validation that meant I was worthy of being chosen. Being chosen was so much more important to me than choosing.

Even as I identified my skills, saw clearly the way I stood out, excelled in school and my career, and was chosen to be a wife, I still fell into the same traps of insecurity, and I often resorted to focusing on my weight, body image, and what else I needed to do to become enough.

Understanding things at a mental level yet only seeing yourself as others see you—even if it's with approval—isn't being settled in your own home. You aren't grounded in who you are until you truly accept everything about yourself and know in the depth of your heart and soul that your biggest responsibility is to be the one you come home to. That doesn't mean we can't be in marriages, partnerships, careers, or friendships. It means that we don't lose ourselves when we do because we have created, and tended to, our own inner home.

We don't need to build our home because it's protective or because that's what people with high self-esteem do, although both of those things may be true. We need to build our own home because it's the only place that will make us happy. It's the only place we can go where we will be the priority 100 percent of the time. The home within is the place where we heal, grow, accept, and nurture ourselves. It's the source of our ability to step fully into life rather than sitting on the sidelines.

Chapter 3
Body Image

A distorted body image and preoccupation with perceived flaws in body shape were common with both of our eating disorders. However, Body Dysmorphic Disorder (BDD) is a separate diagnosis from anorexia and bulimia. According to the Mayo Clinic website, BDD involves preoccupation with perceived flaws in one's appearance, or seeing flaws that can't be seen by others. Neither of us were formally diagnosed with BDD. In our research, we found medical papers detailing differences and similarities between BDD and eating disorders, and they debated whether cross-diagnosis of these disorders is appropriate.

While the number of women with a shared understanding of eating disorders we've encountered has been relatively limited, there's never been a shortage of women who can relate to our struggle with body image.

A blog post titled "11 Facts About Body Image" on DoSomething.org, cites the following statistics on body image from multiple sources. Following are four stand-outs.

1. Over 90 percent of females don't like their bodies and turn to some sort of dieting in an effort to attain their idea of an ideal body.
2. The percentage of women who naturally have the "American" body conveyed by media is about 5 percent.
3. Nearly 60 percent of college-aged females feel pressured to maintain a specific weight and size.
4. Per a survey, two-fifths of women (and one-fifth of men), regardless of gender, age, marital status, and race, said they would consider cosmetic surgery.

Alayna

I remember the day I was told that my eyes didn't work anymore; it was a traumatic and confusing day. I wore prescription contacts, and yet someone was telling me I didn't see correctly. Excuse my language, but what the fuck? That someone was my dietitian. Anyone who works with a dietitian understands that it's a love-hate relationship. She was the only one who truly understood the physical *and* mental aspects of my eating disorder, which is why it was love-hate. I loved that someone got me, but that made her the biggest threat to my eating disorder. She knew how to manipulate it and get inside my head. I often spent our forty-five-minute sessions staring at her and nodding while she explained my eating disorder in depth in her Charlie Brown teacher voice and revealed things I didn't know about myself (like how my eyes didn't work).

Apparently, there's an issue where if you constantly look at yourself in mirrors, you stop seeing yourself objectively. My dietitian described body dysmorphia in much more depth, but all I could understand was that she accused me of having bad eyes. She pissed me off, quite frankly, and I refused to believe her. I saw what I saw in the mirror every day: a girl with way too much extra fat in all the wrong areas.

I often imagined that I could just chop off the fat from my hips, stomach, inner thighs, cheeks, and underarms. Sometimes I even tried. My polka-dotted crafting scissors became my surgical scissors. I liked to scratch them along my hips, pretending I was cutting off my fat. I'd cut deep enough to leave a red scratch for a couple of days. It often made me cry when I was done because I felt pathetic.

One morning I was having bad social anxiety before school, so I walked to the mirror to pick out a body part to be my victim of punishment. I chose my cheeks because I thought they looked too puffy. So, I took my scissors and cut a long scratch starting at my cheek bone and ending near my dimple.

Mom asked me, "How did you get a scratch on your face, honey?"

"Oh, I was petting Paco [our ten-pound cuddly lap-dog], and he got excited and scratched me."

The guilt I felt for lying to my mom was always the worst pain. I exposed my relationship with my scissors to my therapist a few days after the first time, and she nodded with pursed lips and closed eyes. It obviously pained her to hear what I was doing, but it was also obvious that it wasn't the first time she'd heard of such things. I can look back now and see that this was a moment when I became aware that I wasn't alone.

But as long as my eating disorder was still in charge of my thoughts, body dysmorphia was a concept I'd continued to reject. Since I was antisocial and isolated by choice, I didn't have anyone to tell me how I truly looked. So, I had to trust my own judgment, and I was an unreliable source. My brain and my body were no longer on the same page. My brain said that I didn't deserve to eat, while my body screamed for food, but the more my brain ignored my body, the more I lost my hunger cues.

Eventually, I decided to ask my mom what she thought I looked like. I was painting a picture of an ice cream cone (unironically) in the corner of our house that had the most natural lighting and kept me warm and cozy. I was lost in my painting when I heard my mom's gentle footsteps creak over to me and stop right in front of my canvas.

I looked up and she asked, "Alayna, what is your end goal with all of this exercise and dieting?"

I wasn't prepared for this one. I responded with the truth, which I thought was a good thing.

"I don't really have a goal . . . I guess I'll just stop when I'm satisfied with the way I look."

Her expression changed dramatically. In that moment, she'd realized that if her beautiful daughter wasn't happy with how she looked right now, she probably never would be.

My lovely mother said, "I don't want to say the wrong things, but, honey, you're very thin now."

I refused to accept her observation because I believed I was in control of the way I looked, and I saw myself more often and more thoroughly than anyone else.

From that point on, my parents avoided making comments about the way I looked because they were aware it was a dangerous way to approach an eating disorder. And they realized it didn't have an effect on me anymore.

I loved being called thin. One day I was doing yoga in my family room, wearing a sports bra and yoga pants. Nathan was on his way down the stairs, and he looked down into the family room. He told me in a semi-whisper that he could see my spine. His expression and the voice he used still haunts me today. It was the nicest way he could find to say that I looked sickly.

Fast-forward to the present day. I just had a conversation with my mom about body dysmorphia. I've always been curious about why my friends never said anything about how dramatically my body had changed. I told this to my mom, and she responded that several parents, teachers, and family friends frequently expressed their concern for my weight loss. Immediately, I felt proud. Even though I'm recovered now, my eating disorder brain still likes to react to things. It says, "Wow, see, people paid more attention to you when you were thin." And I'm able to say, "Kindly fuck off" to that voice now. But the fact that my *recovered* self still felt a moment of pride for past comments about my body makes me appreciate that people didn't comment to me about my weight loss when I *wasn't* recovered.

If my friends had commented on my body, it would have fed my eating disorder. If someone close to you is struggling with an eating disorder, my number one tip is, "Never comment on their appearance." It's OK to reassure them that they're beautiful or handsome, but avoid specific comments about their bodies because the mind has a unique way of twisting words. Well-intended words may be received and then manipulated in a harmful way.

On another note, when people who weren't close to me expressed their concern, it actually scared me in a good way. For example, one fall day I was running through my neighborhood, and my neighbor—a man that could be my grandpa—was outside in his driveway. I must have looked pretty sickly because he shouted my name while I was running fairly rapidly past his house. I stopped, startled. He looked at me like I was a homeless puppy and said, "Honey, you're looking very thin. It wouldn't hurt ya to put on some holiday weight."

For the rest of my run, I contemplated his words, and for the first time I thought that he could be right. Maybe I didn't see myself correctly. Expressing concern for someone you're not necessarily close with might be the most authentic expression of love you can give.

I'd like to say a few words about the Shiny Demon. This character is a decorative item that's completely irresistible. He grabs your attention when you're walking down the streets past stores.

He says, "Hey! Don't forget to look at me before you leave the house!" and, "Hey! Make sure your body hasn't changed since the last time you looked at me!" You can probably guess who The Shiny Demon is. He's the mirror.

I owned a Shiny Demon that hung on my closet door for several years. I loved him. He always had my back. I put a lot of trust in him. I let him decide whether I could eat or not, what I could eat, how much I could exercise, whether I could go out, and if I was worthy of attention. Needless to say, I was clingy with him. Those who loved me the most and wanted me to get better decided it was a good idea for me to break up with my Shiny Demon.

One morning I woke up and he was gone, probably stashed somewhere in the storage room in the basement. I couldn't rely on him anymore. Taking down my mirror wasn't my choice, but after my mom did it, I was shocked at how frequently I looked over where the Shiny Demon once hung. I even had a whole routine dedicated to the Shiny Demon: face him, stand with feet hip-width apart, feet together until inner thighs touched, bend slightly forward to give myself a thigh gap, straighten back up, lift up shirt to check abs and waist, pinch the fat, turn to the side, suck in to see my ribs, pull shirt back down, walk away with shoulders slumped.

Taking away my mirror was one of the biggest symbolic steps in my recovery. Although there are Shiny Demons EVERYWHERE, taking away the one I viewed most made me realize that what I was doing wasn't practical. There's no way anyone's body changes so much in ten minutes that they actually need to look in the mirror to check.

I still have trouble resisting the Shiny Demon's temptations. Sometimes I still lift up my shirt and check my stomach. I still pose in the mirror trying to find my best angles. But I don't allow these mirror checks to dictate the way I treat my body. In fact, the mirror is sometimes a confidence booster for me now, as it should be for all of us. My favorite thing to do in the mirror is dance. I know it sounds silly, but next time you're listening to your favorite songs, give it a try.

Another way the mirror became a friend was through affirmations. You might've heard of self-affirmations before, and you've probably heard that they're empowering. I heard that for years, but never did anything with that information. One day, I was in the car feeling down, and I remembered my dad telling me how effective self-affirmations were, so I finally tried it. I have a mantra now that I repeat to myself while I'm driving or standing in the mirror getting ready. *I'm smart. I'm kind. I'm beautiful. I'm strong. I'm honest. I'm grateful.* Even though I'm not always those things, after I repeat the sequence about five times, I legitimately believe them. Try it!

Body Image

Melissa

The first time I was exposed to the concept of body dysmorphia was when I watched the movie *The Best Little Girl in the World.* It was 1981, and I was thirteen years old. The character with anorexia, Casey Powell, became overwhelmed at a party and went in the bathroom. As she dug into her purse, she looked up at the mirror over the sink. As the camera focused on the mirror, we saw what she saw—her face stretched wide like a reflection in a funhouse mirror.

The reflection I saw in my parents' mirror that day in first-grade was a distortion. I saw big and fat, when by all accounts—including photos—I was small for my age. When I looked at those girls in the hospital who had tubes in their nose, I saw myself as fat. When I learned the definition of body dysmorphia, I prayed that was the explanation for what I saw in the mirror.

These days I neither question what I see nor look at myself in horror or with great fear, but I do find myself falling into the trap of focusing on one particular body part with judgment. Visually dissecting the body in this way has been part of diet culture for decades. In the mid-1980s there was a "pinch an inch" television commercial promoting a brand of cereal. If you were able to pinch an inch of fat on your belly, you needed their cereal to lose weight. In this advertisement, people pinched their own bellies and those of family and even coworkers. It was a horrifying concept that someone might size you up visually, then grab an inch of your belly to confirm for you both that it was time for a new cereal.

Untold fortunes have been spent on exercise equipment and beauty products that target those cellulite-speckled thighs, chin waddles, flabby arms, sagging butts, and cushion-like abs. And, of course, breast augmentation or reduction. A recent focus on creating puffy lips by the beauty industry takes the cake for me (pardon the expression). What's wrong with our lips? There's nothing wrong with our lips, people. Your lips aren't going to a party. Likewise, your chin waddle isn't marrying your sweetheart. Your butt isn't going to the prom. It's all of you that enters a room.

When we take pieces of ourselves out of context and apply arbitrary standards for what's acceptable, we're losing ourselves. Not just our souls, but our actual selves. The whole body, the big picture. The lips surround our teeth and are part of our face connected to our neck (waddle or not), and so on. This is a case where the whole is truly greater than the sum of its parts.

Questioning is a strategy I use when I find myself evaluating how much money or time I need to spend to bring a specific piece of my body up to the latest beauty standards. I learned this from reading the work of Byron Katie. When we find ourselves distressed about a thought, Katie recommends asking ourselves four questions:

1) Is it true?
2) Can I absolutely know it's true?
3) How do I react when I believe that thought?
4) Who would I be without that thought?

Then, to drive the concept home, she recommends turning the thought around. It's helpful to write out your answers. Let's try it with my belief about what my lower abdomen should look like.

At the time of this writing, I'm approaching my fifty-third birthday and I have what many women refer to as a pooch. There are days when I really hate it. I suck it in as I look in the mirror and marvel at how much better I'd look if that part of me didn't stick out.

Thought: My lower abdomen shouldn't stick out.

1. **Is it true?** Yes, women who are disciplined have flat stomachs. I should be disciplined enough to have a flat stomach.
2. **Can I absolutely know it's true that my stomach should not stick out?** No
3. **How do I react when I believe that thought?** I get angry at myself for not being more disciplined with my eating and exercise. I feel anxious. I am tense and crabby.

4. **Who would I be without the thought that I should have a flat stomach?** I'd be less stressed out when I look in the mirror. I might even like the way my body looks.

Now, turn the thought around and see if the turnaround is as true as your original distressing thought.

Possible turnarounds with rationale:

1. **My lower abdomen *should* stick out.** Maybe at this age, this is what bodies do.
2. **I should *not* be disciplined enough to have a flat stomach.** Maybe the amount of discipline (time and effort) needed for me to have a flat stomach would take away from more meaningful pursuits.
3. **I should be disciplined enough to *not* have a flat stomach.** This one really resonates with me. This would mean letting go of allegiance to an arbitrary beauty standard.

Each of these turnaround statements could be as true as my thought that my lower abdomen shouldn't stick out. Going through this exercise, which Katie refers to as "The Work," brings my anxiety down and chips away at the beliefs diet culture has instilled in me.

The next time you feel compelled to rush out and buy the latest lip-plumping serum, consider the wise words of the

Soothsayer (a goat) to the villain in *Kung Fu Panda 2,* "The cup you choose to fill has no bottom."

There will always be a body part in the beauty industry's limelight. And the way each part is framed as "perfect" will be constantly changing. The butt that was supposed to be small and compact for decades is now being surgically padded. One thing is for sure: diet culture is not going away, so question your critical thoughts and give yourself some grace.

Chapter 4
Thin or Small Equals . . .

Alayna

Barbie has it all. She's got it. The thing we all want: true security in herself. At least that's what I pictured all my life. Allow me to give you a peek at Barbie's real life—if she were a live human. She'd be five foot nine, have a thirty-nine-inch bust, an eighteen-inch waist, thirty-three-inch hips, and a size three shoe. She'd have to crawl on all fours, and she'd fit the criteria for anorexia.

First of all, I hate that there has to be *criteria* to have an eating disorder, but that's for another book. So, let me ask you some things. Do you believe that Barbie's thinness and perfect body give her security? Do you believe that if you could just achieve that perfect figure, then you'd finally be complete? Just five fewer pounds would give you all the confidence in the world? I did, and I want you to know that I don't blame you for believing any of this bullshit either. It's shoved in our faces every waking hour of our lives.

I always think of the image of an angel and a devil on each shoulder to describe what it feels like to have an eating disorder. The first time I realized that my eating disorder thoughts weren't my own was when my dietitian used the personification method from the book *Life Without Ed*. In this book, Jenni Schaefer personifies her eating disorder using the name Ed. I thought my dietitian was crazy at first, but I soon understood why she was calling my eating disorder by another name. It was almost like treating my eating disorder as multiple personality disorder, and it worked. Using the name Ed allowed me to separate myself from his control for the first time. Although I didn't want to give him up, admitting that those thoughts weren't my own gave me a glimpse of freedom. Even though I was still doing what Ed wanted me to do, I was beginning to recognize that I had my own separate desires.

Ed made me believe things that were unrealistic, like the fact that I should look like the mannequins in Fleet Feet. Fleet Feet is a store for runners, so I'd often go there to get new shoes or running gear. One of the first times I resisted Ed was at Fleet Feet while I was buying running shoes with my mom. I looked at a mannequin and immediately thought, *I wish my thighs had a gap like that.* But all the work I'd done to separate myself from Ed made me take a closer look. I stepped forward and grabbed the tag on the mannequin's shorts: XXS, but still cinched and tied to keep them from falling down. *Is this realistic? Is that the type of body that I should be using as an example? Do I even want that?*

I think it's so silly how companies will try to make people feel good about themselves by making them feel thinner in their clothes. I'm a size XS in one of my favorite athletic clothing company's shorts, but if I go to Target for shorts I usually fit best in a medium or large. Which pair of shorts makes me feel better about myself? The answer used to be the XS, because smaller was better.

I genuinely believed that if I was little, someone would have to take care of me. I wouldn't have to ask for help; it would just be given to me. If I was small, then I wouldn't be expected to be strong. People started calling me "cute" and "tiny," and it was incredible. I always had an image in my head of people holding a more frail version of me. In this picture, I was limp, being cradled like a baby in someone's arms. It didn't even matter whose.

For this reason, the idea of inpatient treatment didn't scare me. The thought of being so thin that I wouldn't be able to do anything for myself anymore was actually appealing. Now, I don't want it to sound like I never got the comfort and attention I needed growing up, because I did. But my rigid personality never allowed people to fully take care of me. I never let anyone in, and I sure as hell never asked for help. So, instead of asking for help and admitting that I wanted comfort, I made myself fragile physically.

I got the attention I was looking for, but it didn't fill me up the way I thought it would. Needing my mom to make all my plates, pack all my lunches, give me all my medicines, and drive me to at least three appointments per week wasn't fun. It did make me realize, however, that she was willing to give me all the support she could—no matter what. And *that*, not the fact that I was physically fragile, is what comforted me.

There comes a point when you realize that thin, small, and fragile isn't what you're actually seeking. Because when you achieve it like I did, it's still never enough. You will always be looking for more, whether it's comfort and care like it was for me, or something else entirely. In fact, at my smallest, I had the least amount of compassion in my heart. My desires were completely selfish. I didn't think twice about how I was affecting the people who loved me.

And believe me, I was affecting people in ways I regret tremendously. I know for a fact that people compared themselves to me. I've even talked to a couple of girls I used to sit with at lunch who told me they felt judged by me because I always had healthier lunches than they did and ate less. I don't know about you, but I don't want to be the girl that others feel judged around.

Another thing that keeps me grounded in my true self rather than my eating disorder self is a series of questions I like to ask myself.

- *Do I want to hate my body for the rest of my life?*
- *Do I want to always be trying to get thinner?*
- *Do I want to be anxiety-ridden every time I go out to eat?*

There's an underlying question beneath all of these: *Is it worth it?* And I'm here to tell you: obsessing over your external body is NOT a worthwhile pursuit. Life is way too short to be wasting your energy on something that will never satisfy you. I dislike using the word impossible, but I use it when I need to. It's *impossible* to starve yourself and love yourself at the same time.

Thin or Small Equals . . .

Melissa

Thin and Small = Safe and Protected

This was my story. I believed that standing out in a crowd was dangerous and that the best way to avoid it was to be little, small, and thin. I was small until I was in seventh grade, then I was a normal size. I was never big. I was of average height and a normal weight, if a little on the thin side. But I was no longer *tiny*.

I now understand that I ultimately wanted to be taken care of, and I internalized the notion that girls weren't capable of taking care of themselves in the long run. They'd eventually need a husband to take care of them, and for that, they'd need to be chosen.

Engulfed in the diet culture of the seventies and eighties, it was very clear to me what could get in the way of being chosen: fat.

The Stories We Tell

Our stories give us something to cling to. An identity. An excuse. Motivation. A script to follow. Every story we choose as our headline is chosen because it explains our behavior, mental state, potential, and success (or lack thereof).

A few of my early headlines were:

- I'm Catholic.
- I'm one of six kids. Five girls, one boy. I'm in the middle.
- My dad is the president of the St. Louis Labor Council.

As trauma inevitably enters a person's life, it often becomes the lead in their story. A few of mine over the years were:

- I'm claustrophobic.
- I have a history of eating disorders.
- I'm the mother of a child with special needs.
- I'm divorced.
- I love to work out.
- I'm a runner.
- I'm a single mother.
- I have a NICU baby. She was born weighing 1 pound, 5 ounces.
- I'm never enough.

I've had headlines crafted around my positive experiences and attributes, too:

- I have an MBA from Washington University.
- I'm a career woman.
- I'm a feminist.
- I'm a writer.
- I was once named one of the most influential business women in St. Louis by the *St. Louis Business Journal.*

Sometimes we combine our stories to make a point, as illustrated by a few of my tried-and-true headlines over the years:

- I'm a twice-divorced mother of two kids, and I drive a minivan. No one will want me.
- I had to divorce my husband when my children were only two and three years old. It's been a hard road, and I've done it alone.
- I'm a single mother of two kids, one with special needs, and I work full time.

Often, stories are assigned to us and we accept them as truth:

- You're screwed up.
- That mouth of yours will get you in trouble someday.
- You're too emotional for that job.
- You're not qualified for the job you're in.

We don't always speak aloud the story that's driving us at a given moment. The stories we tell ourselves hold the most power:

- I'm fat.
- I'm thin.
- I'm sick.
- I'm losing weight.
- I'm gaining weight.
- I'm unlovable.
- I'm not enough.
- I'm not worthy of holding on to.

These aren't called stories because they're embellished or untrue. They're stories because they're concepts, ideals, or past experiences we use to create our current intentions, actions, and beliefs. Our stories keep us from living in the present. They keep us stuck. Sometimes they motivate us to do good things, but that's usually out of fear of not living up to the story. When we act out of fear, we aren't at our best.

Eventually, the story I told others shifted from *I have an eating disorder* to *I have a history of eating disorders.* I let go of most of the behaviors over time and just battled the thoughts as they came up. But the real story I lived by, the one I told myself, was *I'm not enough.*

I grew up believing the story that psychological and physical safety are found in others—in their approval of me and in their choosing me. Thus began my hustle to be enough. I attracted and created situations that reinforced that belief. The thing about stories, especially the ones that we tell ourselves, is that they can be rewritten.

Placing my psychological safety in the hands of another isn't only risky; it never works. Even when they're choosing me or approving of me, there's the anxiety that I'll lose them, that they'll change their minds. Najwa Zebian says it best: "When we build our home in others, we give them the power to make us homeless."

Psychological safety is found within. I feel the peace I'm chasing only when I remember that it exists in me already, and I just need to connect to it. It's not waiting for me down the road when I get a better job, more education, a husband, or pay off my debt. It certainly isn't in an eating disorder or the shape of my body. It's within me now, in this breath.

Try that for a story.

Chapter 5
Be a Lady

Alayna

Be gentle, yet strong. Stand up for yourself, but put others first. Speak up for what you believe in, but not too loud. Don't care what people think of you, but make sure you leave the house looking pretty. Don't wear too much makeup or you're seeking attention; if you don't wear makeup, you don't care enough about your looks. Dress too modestly and you're not cool, but dress too slutty and you're asking for it. You can be an athlete but don't let yourself get too masculine looking. These are some of the many beauty standards that I've felt pressed upon me by culture. I'll admit I'm guilty of complying with them.

You see, beauty standards are simply a part of our culture—and always have been—but they depend on the time period and country you're living in. My pale skin isn't something people consider the most desirable today, but take me back a few decades, and people would be envious. Victorians thought almost nonexistent lips were beautiful, but now women are paying incomprehensible amounts of money for lip injections. My point is, beauty standards are just trends, and trying to keep up with them is a vicious cycle.

I was a major tomboy for a few years of my childhood. I think this was due mostly to the fact that I looked up to my older brother, Nathan. Although I didn't want to admit it, he was my role model and always will be. My way of showing this was by wearing his old clothes, rejecting anything that was pink, and taking pride in being sporty.

We all have that cringey stage of childhood—this was mine. But at the time, I was genuinely confident and didn't think twice about what people thought of my style. I thought I was a badass, to be honest. Others? Not so much, and they started making their opinions obvious.

One thing I appreciate about kids is their brutal honesty. The first time I remember feeling the pressure to be more girly was when a boy in my fourth-grade class was talking about his weight. He was a football player and probably the most athletic boy in our class. I remember him declaring his weight proudly like he was a big shot, but I weighed more than he did. So, thinking I was badass and stronger than this boy, I turned to him and said, "Wow, I weigh more than that!"

A few heads turned and his eyes widened. "I wouldn't be very proud of that," he said.

Ouch. The next day was picture day, and I decided to straighten my hair and have my mom put a little braid in it. I remember standing in Target trying to pick out an outfit and nothing was good enough. I wanted to be comfortable, but now I wasn't sure I could do that since, apparently, I shouldn't be proud of my body. I finally chose a cute purple-and-gray-striped shirt and some comfy capri sweatpants. A little bit girly but still casual. Perfect. I showed up to school feeling extremely uncomfortable in my own skin because I was used to wearing my brother's old clothes. As soon as I walked in the classroom, another boy looked at me and made a disgusted face, saying, "*You* dressed girly?!" Well, shit, did people not want me to be girly? This was the first time I noticed a contradiction in what people expected from me.

I always felt different from my friends because I wasn't into pink dresses. The fact that I was outcast because I wasn't ladylike reinforced the idea that in order to be appreciated, I'd have to be girly. Eventually, I grew out of my tomboy phase, but I still valued being a strong, athletic girl. That is, up until I developed anxiety and depression.

In high school, I was under the impression that boys were only attracted to small girls that weren't too loud—girls who didn't take up too much space in the world. Let me just say for your sake: this is so extremely false, but I believed it with my whole heart.

I've *always* been muscular. My dad said I was built like a Burke (which is his side of the family, consisting of him and his three other brothers). I had broad shoulders and strong thighs, but in high school I decided it was time to change them. In the thick of my eating disorder, I made an ultimate sacrifice: lose strength in order to be as thin as possible. I truly did everything in my conscious power to change my body's structure.

I believed I needed to be more dainty and fragile and overall built like a woman. Here was my image of a woman's ideal build: slim but curvy with no extra fat or loose skin or cellulite or too much muscle, but still toned. Jeez, that's a mouthful. I remember believing that everyone was capable of being healthy and achieving all these ideals if they just worked hard enough. I'd completely disregarded the fact that everyone's body is made entirely differently, and also that we all require extra fat on our bodies to *survive*.

I remember being mad at the fact that I was a girl. Why did I have to have extra fat on me that guys didn't have? Why could my brother eat anything he wanted and not gain weight, while I felt like a single burger transferred straight to fat on my body? And the most frustrating question: why did I have to be so sensitive?

You'll hear me say this a lot, but an eating disorder is not *solely* about your body and food. A big part of mine is that I wanted to deny the feminine parts of myself. I heard all the time that women were the sensitive ones—which I do believe we are naturally—but at the time I associated sensitivity with weakness. This was a big reason why I felt like I couldn't share my internal struggles with others; it would show sensitivity and therefore weakness.

Little did I know that being sensitive is a superpower. It doesn't always mean crying over spilled milk; it means being observant and aware of your and others' feelings. I do consider myself sensitive, but it doesn't feel like a curse anymore. The truth is, I'm tough now because of the self-discovery I had to go through, but I'm hypersensitive to those who are struggling mentally. I think it's a beautiful combination.

Be a Lady

Melissa

Why do we have a negative reaction to seeing signs of softness on our bodies? You know what I mean—the dimples, the cellulite, the rolls, etc. Where did that distaste come from? We weren't born with an aversion to these things. Can you remember the first time you heard criticism about your or someone else's body and understood that the message was *intended* to influence you?

According to a 2016 post by the Urban Child Institute, most children under the age of six watch TV for two to four hours each day. This doesn't count the hours when a TV is on in their vicinity. Yet, according to the 2004 American Psychological Association's "Report of the APA Task Force on Advertising and Children," children don't understand that the goal of commercials is to influence them until they are around seven or eight years old. The saturation of cultural messaging starts early.

Advertising is ubiquitous. It's in your social media feed, on podcasts, billboards, buses, scoreboards, bus stops, train stations, trains, airplanes, airports—virtually any commercial property—and of course, magazines, newspapers, TVs, and radios.

Advertising is used to sell products, but it's also used to sell images, concepts, and promises. It crafts an ideal of female beauty and pitches to us that fictitious promised land of perfectionism, as defined by the seller.

Jean Kilbourne began studying the image of women in advertising in 1968, the year I was born. Her poignant documentary *Killing Us Softly* (1979) challenges women to pay close attention to the messages portrayed in advertising. Despite the revelations delivered in this documentary, the objectification of women in advertising has persisted such that *Killing Us Softly* is now a film series that spans three decades.

Kilbourne spotlights the unachievable standards set by altered photography, which is always accompanied by a featured product promising to get you closer to perfection. Women are told they must transform to be beautiful, which always equates to buying something. It's very common that only one part of the woman is featured, essentially dismembering the female body.

Imagery is very powerful. Even an educated woman, who fully understands she's being manipulated, falls prey to the desire to look like the picture, ultimately buying products she doesn't need. We buy into the fantasy that if we just try hard enough, we'll be beautiful, which this culture equates to being lovable.

The twenty-first century has seen a rise in empowering imagery and messaging about women in advertising. One of the more notable ads for me is the #LikeaGirl campaign by Always, which turns the insult of doing something like a girl into a compliment. If you want to be inspired, check out the

"Girl Power in Advertising" collection on the Ads of the World website.

As a midwestern girl steeped in Catholicism—where only boys could be servers at Mass and only men could be priests—and coming of age in a media echo chamber that objectified women, I absorbed the intended message: "Women are inherently less valuable than men, and their value increases when men are pleased with them and when men choose them."

To be a lady was to be agreeable and polite and to make others, especially men, comfortable. I honed my skills of being likable. An off-color joke that made me uncomfortable, unwanted advances from a boss or coworker, a passive-aggressive comment from my teammate . . . I became a master at internalizing, ignoring, or deflecting with the ultimate goal of not making the offender uncomfortable. Men don't choose women who make them uncomfortable.

When we ignore what we feel or believe to make someone else comfortable, we're denying who we are. Instead of using my courage to stop hurtful behavior or to speak the truth to power, I used it for licking my wounds and getting back up with a smile on my face. Proud of my resilience, always revered for my strength. Such a Lady.

But it eventually comes out. It always does—in a sarcastic comment or bit of gossip that leaves me steeped in negative energy. Or it's a painful physical manifestation like a headache. Positive feedback, homecoming queen nominations, business leader awards, and engagement rings cannot fill the hole when we abandon ourselves over and over.

We aren't just victimizing ourselves in this scenario. We're manipulating others to get what we think we want: approval. We're crafting acceptable answers, rather than contributing an original thought. We're anticipating their needs so we can meet them, but not necessarily because we care. It's not altruistic when we behave in a pleasing way to get what we want or gain favor.

Self-deprecation became a close friend of mine. Perhaps ironically, I held her hand when I sensed a *woman* wasn't sure whether she liked me or not. Or if she appeared to be judging my personality based on how I looked. Statements like, "Don't be fooled, I'm a hot mess!" spat forth like a nervous tic when I was praised in front of someone else.

Self-deprecation was always the safest alternative to quietly standing in my truth, with both men and women. I never saw it as manipulative—I saw it as making them comfortable with me. But self-deprecation *is* manipulative. I used it to make others comfortable, so I'd be liked and keep my sense of value intact.

When I was in the hospital, part of the curriculum was assertiveness training. As a die-hard people-pleaser who had built my self-worth on being liked, I didn't catch on quickly to assertiveness training. Imagine a little girl wearing her most beautiful pink chiffon nightgown, her mom's high heels, and a string of pearls around her neck that bounces off her hip bones as she shuffles toward you with frosty, purple Tinker Bell lipstick smeared across the lower half of her face. It was like that. I was a little girl trying to carry herself as a confident woman.

Even in the real world, my attempts at assertiveness didn't land well. They often came out as aggressive rather than assertive, or as too many words trying to sugarcoat the one word I was trying to say: no. And honestly, even when my technique was on point, my message wasn't well received. People don't like to be made uncomfortable, no matter how savvy the delivery is. And they certainly don't want to be made uncomfortable by a young girl. Or a woman in the workplace, for that matter.

There's a voice inside each of us that knows how to speak what it wants and what it doesn't. It may not always be eloquent, but it knows the truth. You can attempt to hush it to a whisper, but eventually, it's going to come out.

When I first started brainstorming this chapter, what came to me was a flood of comments made in my presence either about me or another woman, that echoed "Be A Lady." I've divided it into decades so you can see the progression of topics and messages as I've aged.

The 1980s:

- You must be chosen.
- Don't call boys; they must call you.
- You can marry a rich man just as easily as you can marry a poor man.
- Take a shorthand class, just as a backup. You may need to be a secretary.
- Someday, when you get married . . .
- That isn't very ladylike.
- You have no self-esteem, and that's your problem.

- That mouth is going to get you in trouble someday.
- She said you're boisterous and opinionated.
- I told them you were my pretty one, so please make sure you look nice.
- Notable advertisement for a perfume: "I can bring home the bacon, fry it up in a pan, and never never never let you forget you're a man. 'Cause I'm a woman . . . "

The 1990s:

- She's high maintenance.
- Former boss: You must be wearing your baseball bra. It makes them look round, hard, and firm.
- HR: We've talked to him, carry on.
- Client: I'm happy to sign that contract if you meet me for a drink.
- HR director: If you would like to have an affair, I'd be open to it.
- Company owner: We talked to him, carry on.
- Former boss: She's on the Mommy Track now.
- She's too emotional.
- Image is important.
- It's just business.

The 2000s:

- He cheated on you because you weren't enough. You were a bitch. What was he supposed to do?
- You cheated on him because you're screwed up.

Full: Overcoming Our Eating Disorders to Fully Live

- I know you aren't her boss, but you need to tell her that her clothes aren't appropriate for work.
- He's asking you to present to his client because he wants to travel with you, not because you're good.
- You can have it all: motherhood, career, wife. Give them each 100%.
- You're a bundle of contradictions. I just don't know how to take you.
- Don't take it personally; it's just business.

The 2010s:

- I don't know how you do it all!
- Did you forget again? You didn't see the note in the backpack?
- Former boss: Your back hurts? It's probably all the cum that's stuck up there between your shoulder blades. We need to shake that loose. I'm separated from my wife so there would be no harm done.
- HR: He won't be your boss anymore, but he'll still sit across the hall from you. There's no proof that anything inappropriate was said.
- I watch you in these meetings and you're intuiting what to do by reading other people. You don't really know what you're doing.
- She's "top shelf."
- #MeToo has gone too far. Men can't do anything now without being accused of harassment. That's how things were done back then. You can't punish him for it now.

- It's business; it's not personal.
- Lean in.

The 2020s:

- You left him? Who'll take care of you? You're no longer a kid; you need to think of your future. You can't just go out and find another one. You're running out of time.
- She has special needs kids. This job is too much responsibility for someone with kids like hers. I feel bad for her.
- You don't really have the experience or knowledge for this job, so you use relationships and intuition to get by.
- It's women that are keeping each other down. They need to lift one another up! That's the problem here.
- She's never going to retire. She needs memory care.
- She needs a lot of attention.
- You should see the way the consultants pander to her need for attention. We need to have *serious* business-people at the table.
- You're such a good mom. I respect that. But I want a simple life.

This is how the decades of messaging translate in my thoughts when I'm doubting myself or feeling overwhelmed:

Be a lady, Melissa. Be thin, perfect, nurturing, tough, considerate, strong, unemotional, professional, attractive. Remember, beautiful people are hired more often than unattractive people. Don't forget, overweight people have a harder time making it in the business world. I must be thin. I must be chosen. I must not stand out. I must not take up too much space. I must be strong. I must be low maintenance. I'm not good enough. They don't take me seriously. I'm really not smart enough for this. My kids are too needy for me to have a serious job. I need to run. I need to exercise. No more sugar. I need to work out. Start lifting weights. More yoga. Wait to see if he texts first. Don't push, he needs space. Don't be needy. Watch his ego, he needs attention. Be fun, not too serious. Who'll take care of me? Who'll choose me? I'm so tired. I can't keep up. What would I look like if I just let it go and let my body look how it looks when I eat what I want and move when I can? I need Botox. I need filler. Natural beauty is more beautiful. It's more ladylike.

So, how about this . . . FORGET Be a Lady. Join me in my choice to be my messy, loud, scrappy, beautiful voice of truth. We really do get to choose, and I work on choosing it every single day.

Chapter 6
Shame

Alayna

I'll forever be grateful for one person who stepped in when I needed a persistent friend the most. I call her my sister because we grew up across the street from one another and spent nearly every day together. Audrey was the first person who made an effort to get me out of the house. I was at such a low point that I couldn't bring myself to go to her graduation party because it involved social interaction and scary foods. The second my mom told her that I was feeling anxious and depressed, she texted me during her own party and started planning a time for us to hang out. I didn't respond to her messages for weeks until one day she texted, "I'll come pick you up tonight and we can go get FroYo and talk. I miss you."

People like Audrey are direct threats to an eating disorder because they won't back down. She knew who I really was, and she saw right through the eating disorder's secrecy. I was in no way, shape, or form ready to break the rule I had for myself: go as long as possible without showing anyone how I felt. Ah, yes, avoiding vulnerability . . . a classic human response. Vulnerability is the only solution to shame.

Shame consumes all of us at some point in our lives. There isn't a person in this world who hasn't felt shame. And yet, when shame consumes us the most, we think we're the only ones. It's an emotion with nuclear strength. Perhaps the most frustrating part of dealing with shame is that we're never taught how to. As kids, we don't usually witness adults owning their mistakes. So, when we make our first mistakes, it's only natural that we try to hide what we did. At least, this was my experience growing up.

I made up a word when I was about two years old. I used this word like a cuss word, but I mainly used it when I felt like people were laughing at me or embarrassing me. I'd get so infuriated that my little face would turn beet red, I'd curl up my fists, stomp my foot, and say, "PAFA!" That was my way of hiding my shame as a toddler. Saying a word that made me feel strong and authoritative. Of course, this only made people laugh harder because a cute little girl who could barely form sentences was saying her own form of "fuck you!" So, at a young age, I learned to channel my shame into anger and resentment.

I'd never truly learned how to admit to my shame, and it's no one's fault. It was simply something I didn't want to learn. I thought I could go through life without ever having to be vulnerable. The night Audrey picked me up to go to FroYo and talk, I spent the entire day preparing. I was an anxious wreck. I woke up early, went for a run, and dealt with my anxiety by planning my entire day around the FroYo. You see, it wasn't really the FroYo that scared me, it was the fact that someone was going to make me vulnerable, and there was no more avoiding it. But my brain had become so trained to channel my shame into other emotions that I truly thought it was the FroYo that scared me. And yet, it was the small push from a friend that helped me make the decision to go through with the plans. No more quitting. I didn't know it at the time, but this was the first step to breaking the habit of quitting.

I felt like Rapunzel escaping her castle that night because it was like my eyes were opened to an entirely new world. A world where vulnerability was acceptable. I was pretty quiet on the car ride to FroYo, but Audrey's good at talking, so I felt less pressure. What really made me open up for the first time was when we sat down with our dessert and she asked, "So, how are you *really*, Alayna?" It was the way she tilted her head and opened her eyes real big, like a sad puppy, that made me feel like she could see into my soul. She proceeded to break down my walls one by one until I finally got past the "I'm good, how are you!" fakeness. I told her I had anxiety, that I didn't feel like I had friends, and that I just wanted to lie in bed. Of course, I felt pathetic and like a failure after spilling my guts to her. But, after a pause, Audrey started sharing some struggles she'd gone through in the past, and I was no longer alone.

That night taught me a very important lesson: if you're vulnerable with people, they'll feel comfortable opening up to you. Vulnerability is quite literally a gift that keeps on giving. People *want* to help. Let them.

Scrolling and scrolling and scrolling and double-tapping and zooming in. Those of you on social media know it's toxic most of the time. But I think it's worth noting that in the past few years, there's been an incredible world of vulnerable people on social media. Within the few days after I hung out with Audrey, after a long couple of months of no online contact, I decided to plug back in to social media. To my surprise, people with platforms opened up about their everyday struggles. I even found a bunch of women and teenagers who were open about struggles with eating disorders and body image. Turns out it's extremely common for people to be vulnerable on social media. Who knew?!

I was a girl obsessed with vulnerability. The more I opened up little by little, the more the opportunities to spill my guts came up. I became so good at being vulnerable that oftentimes I couldn't stop myself. It got easier and easier. The point is that I had to start small. I started with telling my parents, then therapists, then Audrey, then a few grade-school friends, then girls in group therapy, then some high school friends, then social media. Then I started giving talks at retreats, and after that, I literally told anyone who had the time to listen. Admitting to your shame takes a whole lot of fucking courage, so don't think I'm trying to promote something that's easy. It's gonna take work. But it's one of the most freeing acts you'll ever experience.

I also want to share something my dad told me one night. I was having a depressive episode, lying in bed with the lights off and staring at my chandelier with tears dripping slowly down my cheeks. My dad has a way of saying the right things. He crawled into my room on all fours like he used to when I was a kid to make me laugh. I knew he was coming up the stairs when I could hear him making the sound of a horse's hooves hitting the pavement: Clack, Clack, Clack. When I was little, I couldn't help but smile and feel giddy as his clacking got closer to my room. He pushed the door open with his head and neighed like a horse, to let me know he had arrived. But this time, I didn't even smile or look in his direction. So, he sat in the gray spinny chair in my room across from my bed in silence with me for about ten minutes.

After what felt like a year, my dad said, "Let me tell you something about baseball players."

Ummm, OK, Dad, this is no time for dad jokes.

He continued, "In Major League Baseball, what's a pretty good batting average?"

I shrugged, still hiding half my face under my covers.

"One in four hits is pretty good."

Crickets . . .

"You know what the funny thing is? The best hitters aren't thinking about their average. They're trying to hit the ball every single time they're up to bat."

I was starting to see where my dad might be going with this weird intro.

"Alayna," he said as he leaned forward, "your failures aren't worth the worry. Just keep getting up to bat."

Getting up to bat again and again is much easier said than done, but the way my dad simplified how I'd been feeling gave me a glimmer of hope. Maybe I could help myself after all. I didn't take action right then and there, but that's not the point. The point is, I used this baseball analogy as a reminder that it didn't matter anymore how ashamed of myself I'd become. The only thing that mattered was how I'd deal with my shame.

So, how do I deal with shame today? I have a new rule for myself: if I fall (literally or figuratively) then I must admit it out loud and use it as motivation to do better. Shame is normal, and it may be healthy to feel it, but it's unhealthy to hide it. I choose to practice my rule in small situations, so that when bigger instances of shame come up, I'm ready to deal with them.

For example, just the other day I totally followed the wrong directions to go eat breakfast with my friends. At first, I lashed out at my boyfriend who was in the passenger seat for not telling me I was going the wrong way. But I caught myself and chose to admit to my shame by saying, "I'm just embarrassed that I'm bad at directions." And saying that one sentence made me laugh and realize there was no reason to hide my shame.

You aren't alone in your shame. You can say you're embarrassed. You can say you messed up. That one act of speaking it will make life a whole lot easier.

Shame

Melissa

I grew up in a Roman Catholic family and went to Catholic schools for primary and secondary education. In grade school, we went to Mass three days a week plus Sunday. The ritual of Mass was comforting. Stand, sit, kneel, sing, pray aloud, pray silently, walk up the aisle, walk back to your pew. And then there was the music. We seemed to rotate through the same fifteen hymns at Mass for the entire time I was Catholic, and while this was the source of many eye rolls, it did annoy me when there was a song I didn't know how to sing. I loved the music, and it's my favorite part of every funeral. I guess the bar is low in that situation, but music brings a sense of peace and belonging for me. It feels like home.

Aside from a few families who were friends of my parents when they were growing up, our social lives centered around our parish. In addition to school and Sunday Mass, there were fish frys, church picnics, and Catholic youth sports leagues. I identified with being Catholic so much that when I was young I thought the kids who went to public school were called "Publics." When I reflect back on my childhood I feel so much gratitude for that community, and I remain connected to many of those families through social media and my family members who still live in that town and go to that same church.

The flip side of my Catholic experience was that I took the doctrine quite literally. Four days a week I was reciting prayers that stated, "Lord, I'm not worthy to receive you . . . " I internalized the concept of original sin—that I was tainted from the first breath I drew and predisposed to sin. Not only was I called to be vigilant with my behavior but also my thoughts. Impure thoughts were sins against God. There were mortal sins—you will burn in hell if you don't make it to confession before you die—and venial sins—you won't go straight to hell but don't let those accumulate! And you didn't actually have to *do* anything, just thinking about the damned behavior was equally offensive. My sensitive nature and perfectionistic personality didn't handle this well.

The Act of Contrition, a prayer that's said aloud by the confessor as part of the confession process, ends with, " . . . I firmly resolve with the help of Thy grace to sin no more and to avoid the near occasion of sin." We Catholics were shooting for perfection. My Catholic school would hold confession at least twice a year beginning in second grade, so by the time I was in seventh grade, I'd gone to confession at least a dozen times.

My failure to stay sin-free for more than a few hours after exiting the confessional led to an obsessive-compulsive response that was very disturbing to me in the moment, and hilarious to my sisters (and me) when I finally confessed it to them. I was so determined to keep my thoughts pure—that was the trickiest part of this whole sin thing—and stressed myself out so much, that as I walked back to the pew from the confessional, I'd accidentally say in my head, "Damn, shit, suck, fuck."

It makes me laugh as I type it, but it was a burden to have sin on my soul less than thirty seconds into my new chance at being a good person. And yet, it was a relief. I'd already lost at perfection, so I could go back to doing my best.

I held on to the shame of being tainted with sin and thinking impure thoughts. Shaming myself became its own sacred ritual. This grew to include shame for my body taking up space, its imperfections, and the need for touch. I believed that shame would keep me humble and motivate me to do good things. In reality, shame threatens our ability to thrive. It leaves us feeling unworthy and renders us listless and depressed or driven to change something about ourselves—all so we can be lovable, rather than because we want that change.

The Struckhoff family home in the Saint Charles Historic District was built in 1890. It was two stories, plus a walk-in attic and an addition to the back of the house that served as the workshop for the family upholstery and drapery businesses. The house was situated on one-third of an acre, surrounded by a white picket fence. The home wasn't fancy, and the entry hall was often narrowed by rolls of fabric that lined the walls, waiting their turn to transform into something functional.

There were two dogs and four kids in the family—and almost always a few extra people. Everyone was welcome at the Struckhoff house, and it was come-as-you-are, day or night—the doors were always unlocked. For that reason, it was the best house in town.

Adam and I started "going together" in seventh grade. In my mind's eye, I can still see him seated in the first desk of the row next to the window in his blue pants and white shirt, legs crossed at the ankles, elbows on the desk, thumbs supporting his chin, five fingers standing at attention on each side of his mouth to project his whisper toward me while preventing others from reading his lips or hearing his words. "Will you go with me?"

Of course, this was all preordained by Adam asking Debbie to find out if I was interested, and Debbie passing back my affirmation. This was middle school, people. Risk-taking was life-threatening.

Standing at the front of my row of desks, books cradled in my left arm, my right hand hanging by my side and wrapped around the handle of my flute case, I smiled, nodded, and floated out of the room toward band practice.

To be clear, we were going nowhere. We were twelve. We didn't even change classrooms during the school day. But that was how we professed our special relationship status in 1980. Every night for the next two years, Adam called me at 6:30. Everyone in the Kelley household knew they had to be off the phone by 6:30, so Missy could talk to Adam. Technically, I guess you could say we were going to the phone together.

This was the first of many times Adam would ask me to be his girlfriend, in whatever the vernacular of the day, as we would break up and get back together countless times through high school and our early college years. Growing up was terrifying to me, and Adam grounded me. He was always on my side, and even when we were broken up, the bond was strong.

The night before I went into the hospital for the first time, I was with Adam, and we were both crying. He looked at me through watery green eyes, and all sixteen years of him expressed this most profound truth about love: "I'm with you, even when I'm not."

He understood me better than I understood myself, and he loved me deeply. Of course, we were kids, and it was love, so as much as we would love one another over the eight years of our on-and-off romantic relationship, we would also hurt each other in the way only a first love can.

There was a party at Adam's house in the fall of eighth grade. We snacked in the kitchen, slung sarcasm in the TV room, and gossiped in the hallway. As the evening wore on, we self-sorted into two rooms. The couples in the room with the light off, and everyone else in the room across the hall, presumably with the light on. I wouldn't know.

"Air Supply" crooned from the boombox in the dark room as couples slow-danced and kissed. For most of us, it was our first long make-out session. At this age, there weren't many opportunities for affection other than a quick kiss behind the gym before a car pulled up. Parties were the love lifeline, and they were few and far between.

Slow dancing involved rocking side to side, to no apparent beat, while the girl's arms circled the boy's neck, and the boy's arms circled the girl's waist. No skill required. Just raging hormones. Invariably, the boy would test his luck at unlocking his hands and rubbing them up the girl's back and slowly down toward her bottom, retreating quickly up the back in response to any tensing or flinching.

Confident in the established safe zones on the back of the body, he'd inch his hands toward the sides of her body, resting them around her ribcage. Periodically, eyes would creep open, darting around the room to see what everyone else was doing and who might be watching.

All good.

Nothing to see here.

Just slow dancing.

Rocking side to side.

Kissing.

"Lost in Love and I don't know why . . . "

And then, in one quick move, leaving no time to chicken out, the right hand moved from the rib cage to the breast.

A gasp.

A squeeze.

Intense kissing.

Eyes open. Check the group.

Carry on.

When we could hear our friends in the other room saying good-bye and heading down the hallway toward the door, we knew it was time to turn on the light, exit the room, and act like nothing happened. As I crossed the threshold, I saw my friend Denise, and in an instant those warm, tingly feelings were replaced by a splash of prickly, cold shame.

I lay awake that night obsessing over what Denise and the other kids thought of me. I thought about my mom and how ashamed she'd be if she knew I let Adam touch me (over the clothes). I was disgusted with myself.

I got distracted by flashbacks of the warm kisses and closeness to Adam. Reliving every single minute of every single song. Then I'd catch myself and feel the rush of shame again.

I deserved to be punished, so I broke up with Adam the next day. He was confused and devastated. I didn't want to do it, but more than that, I didn't want to be bad.

Damn. Shit. Suck. Fuck.

In *A Theory of Human Motivation*, Abraham H. Maslow presents a hierarchy of needs, expressed as a pyramid, to explain what compels us to act. This isn't intended to be a list of what humans must have in order to survive or thrive, rather it's a theory about what motivates human behavior. There are other determinants of human behavior besides motivation, like social, cultural, and situational circumstances. But all behavior is motivated.

I see two important premises of Maslow's theory relative to shame:

1) A given need-state not only affects our short-term motivation, it also affects our philosophy of and outlook on the future. For example, the chronically starved man believes that a life in which there's plenty of food is all he needs to be happy. He perceives freedom, love, and community feeling as whimsy compared to a life where food is plentiful.
2) Any of the physiological needs and the resulting behaviors can serve as channels for other needs. For example,

the girl who thinks she's hungry may actually be seeking comfort rather than nutrition, and conversely, it's possible to satisfy the hunger need by drinking water or smoking cigarettes (Maslow 1943, 5). So, while our physiological needs may seem discrete, they can overlap with other needs.

Maslow's Hierarchy of Needs

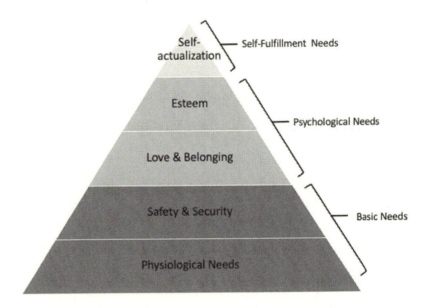

The needs at the base of the pyramid are the physiological needs that must be met to stay alive. These have the greatest influence on our actions or behavior. If one is starving, all capacities are directed in the service of satisfying hunger. "Capacities that are not useful for this purpose lie dormant, or are pushed into the background" (Maslow 1943, 6). The urge to buy a Jet Ski™ or write the great American novel is either abandoned or forgotten.

Once the physiological needs are satisfied, a new set of needs emerge—those of safety. In our modernized society, our safety needs are generally satisfied and aren't usually an active motivator for behavior. For example, except in unusual or extreme circumstances, we don't fear death from wild animals when we're heading to the kitchen for dinner. Of course, there are situations where safety could be our primary motivator. Driving home in a blizzard, our primary motivator for putting the phone in our purse and two hands on the wheel could be safety. In circumstances of chronic abuse in the home, the need for safety may jump to the forefront in motivating our actions.

Right smack in the middle of the pyramid is love and belonging. While this need may seem less critical than the basic needs, remember that when the other need-states are satisfied, we're catapulted to the next level (need-state) of the pyramid, and that next need becomes the source of all motivation. This explains why we find ourselves desperately wanting a boyfriend, or friend group, or to fit in at work so much that we sometimes do things we don't really want to do or that we're ashamed of later.

Satisfying this need for love and belonging is the springboard to the motivation that drives the very best of what life has to offer: self-actualization. When we feel connected to others, whether it's a church group, a sports team, or just one single person, our motivation shifts to accomplishing things that make us proud and explore the bounds of our potential.

Without a sense of love and belonging, we're just doing what needs to be done to keep ourselves breathing and protected.

Brené Brown says shame is a state of feeling that one isn't worthy of love and belonging because of something they did, a characteristic they have, or one they're lacking. When we hold onto shame, it's impossible to satisfy the need for love and belonging. In this way, my eating disorder was one long hustle to become worthy of love, friends, popularity, and a husband.

My shame was fed by my perception of how my body measured up compared to others, height/weight charts, BMI calculations, and clothing sizes. My shame motivated me to diet, run, cover up my body with clothes that were too big, and obsess about my body to the extent that I couldn't imagine a future for myself.

The summer before my senior year of high school, I went to a leadership camp where it seemed everyone else was having fun and thinking about their futures. I cried for the first week. Not because I was homesick but because I didn't belong in this place where smart, happy, motivated people designed happy futures. We took tests to figure out which careers we may be suited for, and I dissociated from the entire process. Every time I tried to imagine myself as an adult going to work, I saw a large, white, foggy room. A nothingness. I believed I wouldn't live that long, and if I couldn't get my body closer to perfect, I didn't want to.

I believe that learning what to do when you're in the midst of what Brené Brown refers to as a "shame storm" can be transformational for everyone, especially people who struggle with eating disorders and body image. There are many approaches, you just have to find something that works for you in a given situation. The things that have been helpful to me are rooted in the work of Marsha Linehan (Dialectical Behavior Therapy), Brené Brown, and Byron Katie. What works in one situation may not work in the next, so it's nice to have a menu of options. The following are three items you can add to your menu.

Exercise One: Check the Facts. (DBT)

Dialectical Behavior Therapy was created by Marsha Linehan to help people who were considered unfixable, like the chronically suicidal. It's a therapy framework that provides practical tools to address issues that underlie the feelings that lead to the desire to self-harm. There are four modules: mindfulness, distress tolerance, emotion regulation, and interpersonal effectiveness.

From the emotion regulation module, "Check the Facts" is a tool that helps me manage my shame. Here's an example:

1) Identify the emotion you want to change. *Anxiety mixed with shame.*
2) What is the situation that led to this emotion? *I texted the guy I've just started dating to ask if he'd like to meet me for dinner tomorrow. It's been a couple hours and he hasn't responded.*
3) What are the thoughts I have about the situation? *He doesn't want to go to dinner with me because he doesn't like me anymore, and it's because of that stupid thing I said the last time we were together, and why didn't I just keep my mouth shut. He's probably trying to decide whether to tell me he doesn't want to go to dinner with me or just ghost me.*

4) Are my thoughts fact-based? Or, am I making assumptions and treating them as truth? *Ummmmm. Well, it's been two whole hours, and I said that stupid thing!*

5) What are the facts of the situation? Just the facts, ma'am. *I sent him a text asking him to dinner, it's been two hours and he hasn't responded. That's all I know to be true.*

When I check the facts like this, I can easily see that I'm making up stories that I can't possibly know to be true, and those stories make me feel anxious and ashamed. This exercise can be combined with the tool offered by Byron Katie.

Exercise Two: Question your thinking. (The Work)

Byron Katie is a spiritual teacher and author who, like Linehan, found herself in an inpatient psychiatric setting that didn't help her. She created what's referred to as "The Work of Byron Katie," or "The Work," which guides us through questioning our thoughts and ultimately accepting exactly what's happening now, in the present moment or situation, with grace and peace in our heart and mind. This concept is similar to "Check the Facts," but I find "The Work" to be a helpful follow-up to that exercise because while checking the facts helps me understand the situation objectively, "The Work" helps me embrace it and see it as my friend and teacher.

Here's how it goes:

1) Notice what's bothering you and write it down. Who are you judging? What are you judging? Be radically honest.

2) Ask four questions: Is it true? Can I absolutely know it's true? How do I react, what happens, when I believe that thought? Who would I be without that thought?
3) Turn it around. Is the opposite thought as true or truer than the original thought?

Exercise Three: Reach out to a trusted confidant and tell your story. (From the work of Brené Brown)

Shame loses its power when it's brought into the light. How many times have you thought something was unspeakable, then finally told someone and realized it didn't sound as bad as it felt? When we share our shameful event with someone else, we starve shame of its food, which is secrecy.

This is the hardest of the three items for me. While I'm like an open book most of the time, the things that feel the worst, the things I'm ashamed of, I like to keep hidden.

I have different people that I tell my shame stories to, depending on the shame event. My friend Leslie is my go-to gal when it's related to a "mother-of-the-year" moment, such as when my two-year-old told my three-year-old, "Put your god-damn shoes on, Wobbie [Robbie]." The only word she said with perfect diction was "goddamn." Darcie is my go-to friend when I feel shame around something that's happened in a relation-ship. There are others, too. One person can't be your every-thing. Just make sure the person is someone you trust for that particular genre of issues, so you don't end up feeling judged and more ashamed after telling the story.

Chapter 7
Perfectionism

Alayna

I'm a little detail oriented . . .

When Grandma Jane came over, we colored; it's what I looked forward to each time she visited. I always watched her coloring strategy in awe as she moved her crayons in a circular motion to leave no obvious coloring lines. Perfect.

"Let's clean up, I'm ready to do something else," my five-year-old self said. Grandma started putting the crayons back in the box. *Oh, God. No. No, no, no.*

"Grandma, NO! They go in RAINBOW order."

I'm a little obsessed with perfecting skills . . .

"Alayna, why don't you come in for dinner? You've been on the trampoline for two hours straight!"

"No thanks, Mom. I still can't do a full twisting back flip."

I'm a little afraid of being imperfect . . .

"Hey, Alayna, what did you get on that math test?"

"None of your business!" That's what I'd reply, even if it was 90 percent.

I'm a little ashamed of not reaching perfection . . .

Perfectionism is part of who I am. My Myers-Briggs personality is INFJ or ENFJ, my enneagram is 1, my Color Code is red, and my sun sign is Pisces. If those don't mean anything to you, just know that even the internet can tell I'm obsessive. It's a blessing and a curse, no doubt. It's a blessing because it means I won't stop until I get the job done and done *correctly*. But it's a curse because it means I'll put my entire life on pause if that's what it takes to accomplish my desired goal.

I did put my life on pause once. As soon as anxiety became a part of my identity, I let it control my passions. The things I loved most were volleyball, fitness training, learning, being creative, spending time with friends, laughing, and being productive. It was no longer enough to simply love things anymore, though; I had to be *the best*. The scary part about trying to be the best is that you can't do it in every area of life. I felt that being anything but the best was a failure.

I don't know about you, but when I fail, I give up. I started giving up on volleyball. Panic attacks became normal during practice and games. At a tournament one time, the other team served the ball to me, and I shanked the ball, destroying my team's opportunity to get a point. *Fail.* This happened two more times consecutively, and by the third time, my heart was pounding so fast I had to hold my chest. At that moment, I went through everything I'd eaten that day to calm me down: *six carrots, one apple, a little bit of peanut butter.* I looked at my parents in the stands and saw their concern. Their faces reminded me that I was a problem, and the panic got worse. So I ran off the court in the middle of the next play, cried on a toilet in a dusty bathroom, and tried to pull my hair out.

Next was academics. I'll never forget the night when I had a history presentation the next day, and I hadn't even started it. Alayna Burke doesn't procrastinate, so this was a shock to everybody, especially my parents. I came home from school, laid in bed for a couple hours, skipped dinner, and finally came downstairs with my laptop in my hands and stared at my parents. What I wanted to say was, "I'm having trouble focusing on my homework because I'm extremely stressed lately, and I feel like my life is falling apart."

What I actually said was, "I can't."

It took about an hour for my parents to get it out of me that I had a group project due tomorrow. I told them about my group members: two girls I'd gone to grade school with. My dad being the productive, practical man that he is, decided that it was a great idea to call their parents and tell them I was having trouble with the project. *That sounds like I'm imperfect, Dad. Never expose my flaws—don't you know that?!* Boom, tantrum thrown on the hardwood kitchen floor. Screaming, crying, and begging him not to call those parents. He agreed, so I calmed down a bit and continued to stare into space with my hungry and tired eyes. After a while, staring gets old.

Tom Burke is not a patient man, but he saw the hurt in my eyes. He took my computer, read over the assignment, and typed for about thirty minutes straight. He finished my project that night, and I got a B on it. Stories like this remind me that sometimes just getting the job done is enough.

Being thin was something I could try to be the best at. I subconsciously knew there'd always be someone in the world who was thinner than me, and as a perfectionist, I liked the fact that I could chase after a goal so extreme. On the outside, I looked like a girl who was healthy and liked to cook her own meals and take care of her body by exercising every day. What people didn't see was that most of the healthy meals I cooked got thrown in the trash, and most of my workouts were filled with anger and hatred of my body. I was never enough for myself. I had a rule: be the thinnest in any given room.

At the doctor's office, I remember comparing myself to a young girl who was probably eight; I was sixteen. I remember being jealous of my dog because he could survive on one meal per day without being hungry for more; he weighed ten pounds. It's crazy how I'm able to look back now and realize that I usually was the thinnest in the room, but I always found something else that I wasn't the "best" at, which completely blocked out the fact that I was getting thinner every day. Every elevator, classroom, fitness studio, and park . . . there was always someone better than me. *FAIL.* I forgot that it's a beautiful thing that everyone has different skills.

I even wanted to be a perfect introvert. What does that even mean? It means I thought that I didn't need other people. Boy, was I wrong! Let me explain a common misconception about introverts. They aren't always shy and quiet, and they sure as hell need social interaction just like extroverts; they just get their energy from alone time. I was an introvert that desperately lacked social interaction. The thing about eating disorders is that they're secretive and isolating. So the combination of me wanting to be the perfect introvert and my eating disorder holding me in the shadows made me oblivious to the extreme torture I was putting myself through. I didn't go out, so how was I supposed to measure if I was the smallest in any given room? That's the most dangerous part—I had only people on the internet to compare myself to. I'll get more into comparison later, but my point is that I got sucked out of reality and couldn't see that I was, in fact, sickly.

You probably wonder how I got over the perfect introvert phase and rediscovered social skills. This is my favorite story. I'm a vivid dreamer, no doubt. My best dreams come when I go to bed without looking at my phone first, but I'm convinced that God plants dreams in my head when he sees that I'm desperate. I was starting my junior year of high school, I was at the peak of my eating disorder, I was at my lowest weight, and I didn't have any sort of social interaction other than with my family. To flesh out the story from earlier, one night I had a dream that I was in a cross-country practice with the girls in my class who ran on the team. I was running through the neighborhood that my school was in, and I couldn't stop smiling and laughing. There was light all around me that looked like one of those scenes from a movie where someone sees a glimpse of heaven. Most importantly, though, I was running right smack in the middle of the group of girls, and I felt light as a feather.

Words don't do this dream justice, but it woke me up in the middle of the night with a jolt. My heart was pounding out of my chest, and I literally woke up smiling in my bed. Here's the exact journal entry I wrote as soon as I woke up from that dream:

8/13/2019   3:00 AM Noisy Mind

I can't stop thinking about cross country.

PROS: keep me in shape, more involved, satisfy curiosity, fun girls, reason to eat

CONS: less free time, haven't been eating

God, I trust that if I pay attention you will reveal what I should do.

The next day was already the second day of tryouts, but it was a no-cut sport. I worked up the courage to text the girls on the team and email the coach to see if they thought I should do it. They were extremely supportive. I went through tryout week and met a girl in my class who I'd never really talked to before.

Running together is probably the most efficient way to make friends because it forces you to go through a struggle together and to occupy each other's minds. That's exactly what we did. Obviously, running burns a lot of calories and was very dangerous for my health at the time, so my dietitian wasn't too happy that I joined the team. But on the other hand, my family and doctors started seeing me smile again and talk about the fun I had at practice. I even went to the state meet that year with my team and discovered running was a talent of mine.

The reason this simple story is my favorite is because it was a time when I didn't put any pressure on myself to be the best. I was just running for the benefit of my mental health. I encourage you to find those hobbies that allow you to work hard and smile at the same time, and you'll find that they will lift you out of the extreme competition you expose yourself to daily.

Perfectionism

Melissa

For my first couple of decades, I believed that life's difficulty level would plateau once I reached a certain milestone. The milestones kept changing and were just far enough in the future that the present moment was filled with a sense of lack. *I'll be happy when . . .* Or, *I'll be happy if . . .*

I held tightly to the belief that I needed to be taken care of and that my job was to be good enough to be chosen. On the few occasions when I found someone with whom I had a true connection, I'd describe it as, "He feels like home." I've spent my entire life working to perfect who I am so that "my room," (myself), would be worthy of someone else's home. This would be the plateau, the part where life got easier.

Zebian's book *Welcome Home* was like truth serum, the last puzzle piece, the last class of the last semester of a college degree. I'm not a room, I'm a house. And I'm the only house that will ever be a permanent home to me. When I live my life as a room looking for a house, I give someone else the power to make me homeless.

I've danced the dance of love and loss many times, which invariably leaves me feeling that I'm just not enough. *Yet. I just need to be more perfect!* Cue hyper focus on exercise, eating, and an obsessive search for the right book or podcast that will help me do life better.

This search for ways to do life better has served me well. I've developed a powerful spiritual practice that's void of religion and doctrine, and it has deepened my empathy and compassion and strengthened my sense of worthiness and belonging. And yet, in one fell swoop, a breakup or rejection can vaporize that growth and leave me desperate to repeat the cycle of perfecting myself, believing I'm a room in search of a home.

I like listening to self-development books while I'm cleaning, driving, or walking. (Don't want to waste a minute—perfection takes time!) *Welcome Home* takes you through the process of creating inner space, boundaries, and tools to support you as you journey through the highs and lows of life. Zebian proposes that all you have and will ever need for emotional security and happiness is within this space, which is compared to a house.

The sweltering sun beat down on me as I walked our new puppy through the neighborhood. I was, for the second time, listening to the chapter on building a foundation, when clarity dawned. The reason my house turns to dust when a relationship ends is because it's built on a foundation of knowledge, not acceptance. Knowledge isn't the same as acceptance. While it's important to know ourselves well, to be aware of who we are, knowledge without acceptance yields judgment, and in my case, the drive for perfectionism.

Acceptance grounds us. It doesn't mean we stop evolving into a better version of ourselves, it means we apply compassion and empathy to that knowledge of who we are, so our actions come from a place of love instead of fear. Acceptance is the opposite of perfectionism. Acceptance is rooted in love, perfectionism in fear.

I was surprised by the volume of research papers that address the impact of perfectionism on mental health: perfectionism and eating disorders, perfectionism and anxiety, perfectionism and depressive disorders, perfectionism and suicidal ideation to name a few. In reading a few of these papers, as well as some popular psychology and even business articles, I learned that it's generally agreed that there are three types of perfectionism:

1) Self-oriented perfectionism: characterized by rigidity, extremely high, self-prescribed standards for oneself, and highly critical, obsessive self-dialogue.
2) Other-oriented perfectionism: expects perfection from others and highly critical of them when they fail to meet these expectations.
3) Socially prescribed perfectionism: driven by the belief that others expect them to be perfect, compounded by fear of criticism and isolation if they don't meet those standards.

I've fallen prey to all three of these traps, and I now easily identify the various forms at work in people around me. Perfectionism, like "a little bit of anorexia" is viewed as a noble characteristic. In job interviews, candidates commonly claim it as a fault. A humble brag, if you will. One business article I came across cited self-oriented perfectionism as a desirable characteristic in employees.

Leading up to the 2020 Tokyo Olympics, which took place in 2021 due to the COVID-19 pandemic, there was much fanfare—really an obsessive focus—about Simone Biles, the twenty-four-year-old American gymnast who was lauded the "GOAT" (greatest of all time). Over the course of her gymnastics career, Simone had taken the athleticism of gymnastics to a new level. As of this writing, Biles is the most decorated gymnast in Olympic history. She has four skills named after her, holds records for most world championship medals, and earned the most gold medals in those competitions. She also holds the most all-around titles from world championships.

As Biles crushed records and repeatedly raked in the gold, she increased the difficulty of her skills. There was much discussion and debate among pundits and analysts over how she was scored relative to other gymnasts because she was performing at a level of difficulty previously unseen. She was in a league of her own. On NBC's *TODAY* show in April 2021, Biles said, "I'm trying to beat myself. That's what motivates me."

Four weeks before the Olympic Cauldron was lit in Tokyo, Japan, Biles won her second All-Around Champion title at the Olympic trials in Saint Louis, Missouri. While the difference in scores between the leaders at gymnastics meets is typically counted in tenths and even hundredths of a point, Biles won the title with a two-point lead over second-place finisher Suni Lee. However, on the second day of the meet she both fell off the balance beam and straddled her legs during a handstand on the bars. "That doesn't happen [to Simone Biles]," the NBC announcer said as Simone made this uncharacteristic mistake.

After the incident on the bars, as she approached her teammates who received her with fist bumps and encouraging words, Simone could be heard saying, "I want to die." The announcers credit her "high standards" for her "over-the-top" remark, rebutting that she's "still the best gymnast in the world."

As the Olympic games approached, the pressure on Biles continued to mount. In a *New York Times* article titled, "Simone Biles and the Weight of Perfection," published the day before the U.S.A. women's gymnastics team competed in the qualifying round, Simone is quoted as saying, "Probably my time off," when asked about the best moment of her career.

Biles was the perfect gymnast, the greatest of all time. She'd had to make up new skills because she'd perfected those available to her at the time, which was unfathomable to her peers. And she wanted it to be over.

After her first vault on the first night of the 2020 Olympic gymnastics competition, Biles withdrew from the meet citing mental health reasons. She later explained that she had the "twisties," which is an extremely dangerous mental block that affects spatial awareness.

On her Instagram, Biles wrote, " . . . I have no idea where I am in the air I also have NO idea how I'm going to land. Or what I'm going to land on. Head/hands/feet back . . . "

Simone walked away from perfection in front of the whole world. For real. She prioritized her health and wellbeing, knowing some people would feel let down by this decision and others would judge her harshly. There were countless social media posts supporting Biles and thanking her for demonstrating the courage to choose her physical and mental health and for

Full: Overcoming Our Eating Disorders to Fully Live

setting an example of how pleasing others isn't something to be done at any cost.

Piers Morgan, a British journalist, begged to differ. The following day, he tweeted his column for the *DailyMail.com*, highlighting this comment: "Sorry Simone Biles, but there's nothing heroic or brave about quitting because you're not having 'fun' – you let down your team-mates, your fans and your country."

Biles didn't back down. Instead, she advocated for mental health awareness for athletes. In a press conference following her bronze medal win on the beam in the apparatus finals several days later, she said, "It [the topic of mental health] should be talked about a lot more, especially with athletes, because a lot of us are going through the same things and we're always told to push through it. At the end of the day, we aren't just entertainment, we're humans and there are things going on behind the scenes that we're also trying to juggle with as well, on top of sports."

And, in a social media post following Piers Morgan's column, Biles said, "We have to protect our minds and our bodies and not just go out and do what the world wants us to do."

No matter which type of perfectionism you're operating under, it's unsustainable and exhausting. If it's the fuel that drives your eating disorder, it's as dangerous as launching yourself off a vault when you can't tell the difference between up and down. Choosing yourself over the subjective and fluctuating standards of perfection takes courage and requires acceptance.

Accepting the limitations of her mind and body, Simone Biles walked away from perfection. Seven days later, she returned to compete on the beam in the individual apparatus finals with a modified routine that accommodated her limitations. Her smile and excitement after she beautifully (and safely) dismounted was worth more than gold.

"A routine that will resonate for years to come," exclaimed the NBC announcer as we watched Simone receive tearful hugs and smiles from her coaches and teammates.

By gymnastics standards, Simone Biles was far from perfect that night. She took bronze. But if there was ever a lesson in the deceit of perfection, it's the story of Simone Biles.

Chapter 8
Control

Alayna

If my eating disorder was a car, control would be in the driver's seat. Above all, I believe the never-ending search for control is what kept me from thinking rationally. I was always very put together, so anxiety and depression made me feel like I was losing my grip on my life. *How could I let myself get this bad?* To ease the anxiety this question created, I subconsciously searched for control.

My therapist called my eating disorder, "a log in the middle of a fast-flowing stream." Safety. It was there when I so desperately needed something to grab on to. The tricky part about grabbing hold of a log in a fast-flowing stream is that once it's safe enough to let go, it takes a hell of a lot of courage to do so, since the log was the very thing that saved you.

That's why letting go of an eating disorder can seem impossible. Because it gives you a sense of control over a part of your life that you need more than anything. For me, controlling my food and exercise kept me sane. But it also made me oblivious to everything else in my life that I was giving up. The truth is, there's pretty much nothing in life you can have 100 percent control over without sacrificing something else. For example, if you want to be completely in control of your work life, you might find yourself sacrificing family time. If you want to always have straight As, you'll probably have to give up some parts of your social life. Giving your all to one thing takes a significant amount of energy. I put every ounce of my energy into making myself thinner. I couldn't even imagine myself having fun anymore.

My life was thin. Thin was my life. I was miserable, but having an eating disorder finally made me feel in control. I was proud of myself for getting "that bad" because I thought it showed discipline. Ladies and gentlemen, that's NOT the kind of discipline to follow. It was the kind of discipline that didn't allow for victory. Or achievement. Or rest.

Controlling my body made me oblivious to the harm I was doing to myself and others. The first time I realized I was being extreme was in a therapy session. My therapist talked about how people with eating disorders, or any form of OCD or anxiety for that matter, often have rules for themselves.

Rules? No way. Couldn't be me.

Boy, was I in for a rude awakening!

She said, "Think of some rules you have for yourself over the next couple of days and write them down." To my surprise, I had a full page within two days. My rules included restrictions on eating times, quantity, form (liquid/

solid), where I ate, and a requirement to compare what I ate with that of others. I brought this list with me to my next therapy session. My next assignment was, "Challenge at least one of these rules." I hadn't really begun to resist my eating disorder yet, so the idea of challenging it made me feel like I was being forced to let go of the log and drown to death.

This is where the infamous meal plan came into play. My dietitian decided that I wasn't getting enough nutrition by just dropping some of my rules. So she wrote out a meal plan that had three meals and about three snacks per day (which, by the way, is perfectly normal and actually ideal). You should've seen my face and felt my heartbeat. This lady was using my control-freak brain against me. It's actually quite genius if you ask me now. My brain saw this meal plan as a chance to be perfect if I followed it exactly. She scribbled it down on a blank piece of paper with a blue pen. She wrote in silence while I waited and struggled. *I thought I wasn't supposed to follow rules?*

I was pissed at my dietitian. God bless her soul for putting up with the sass I gave her every session. "You want me to *measure* the amount of oatmeal I eat?" I asked her sarcastically.

"Precisely," she responded.

"Goldfish aren't even healthy. Why are you making me eat them every day if you're a dietitian that's supposed to help people eat healthy?"

She replied with a smile, "No food is good or bad. We'll work on that."

The meal plan would be my temporary replacement log in exchange for my unhealthy, rigid rules. However, I still had to make the jump to this next log.

Letting go of control is the hardest part. I wouldn't have made the decision to let go bit by bit if it weren't for the glimpses of freedom I started to see. For example, letting go of the no eating out rule reminded me how good my favorite restaurants were. Ditching the time of day restriction around eating made me sleep ten times better and wake up energized. Challenging the no liquid calories rule gave me a newfound love for coffee (with actual creamer and sugar). Giving up control gave me back my life.

I still am, and probably always will be, a control freak, but I know it, and that gives me all the power in the world to keep it . . . well . . . under control.

I encourage you to be spontaneous every once in a while. Maybe you have your whole day planned out today, but something comes up and gets in the way of your perfect plans. Take the opportunity to let go of control. That's something I've been working on recently. Each time a friend texts me with last-minute plans, I take a deep breath and remind myself that spontaneity is a good thing. We could all stand to be a little less attached to our schedules.

Control

Melissa

I was a bed-wetter until I was fourteen. I don't have a great sense of smell, but the scent of urine comes to me with a thought. My parents did everything they could think of to prevent me from wetting the bed. I stopped drinking water after 7:00 p.m., and they'd wake me up and take me to the bathroom several hours after I'd gone to sleep. Sometimes it worked, sometimes it didn't.

I was one of six kids and there was a lot of laundry. Having a kid pee in the bed several times a week had to be overwhelming for my mom, and the longer this went on, the angrier she got. She thought I was being lazy. One time I was so afraid to get in trouble I stripped the sheets and put them in my closet. A couple days later when the sheets were discovered because they stunk to high heaven, I definitely got in trouble.

I couldn't control it. I was so anxious about it and tried so hard that I developed a recurring dream in which I needed to pee so badly that I'd run into the bathroom to avoid wetting the bed. In my dream I'd make it to the toilet just in time to feel that glorious relief of emptying a bladder that was about to explode. The relief would last about five seconds when I'd awake to realize I was peeing all over myself and my sister with whom I shared a bed. I was so ashamed. And it happened over and over. I couldn't control it.

The church picnic was called the "Family Affair," and it was the best part of fall. Every year in late September, the parking lot of the church—which doubled as the school playground—was transformed into a carnival with rides, game booths, and food stands. The third-grade classroom became the bank, the dads the bankers. Those tiny, perforated tickets were worth more than gold to us kids.

The year I entered sixth grade, the Family Affair left an indelible mark on my psyche. Throughout most of grade school, Marie was my best friend. I thought she was perfect. She was so smart and kind and virtuous. She was the youngest of three girls, and her sisters were equally special. Always the best in the class, she was known for being smart and holy. I remember in first grade thinking that maybe she was actually Mary (the mother of Jesus) because she was so good. We spent a lot of time together, and as much as I liked her, I often felt awkward and flawed around her. I knew she accepted me as I was, but I also knew I wasn't as good as her.

Marie and I were in the "Green Monster." That's how I've named it in my memory, but I don't know what the ride was actually called or what color it was. I remember it being like a mechanical seesaw, high in the air, with a passenger cab on each end. The cabs rotated so that when the see-saw lifted us high, the door to the cab faced the sky, and when we came back down, the door to the cab faced the ground. The passengers slid across the cab—all the way to the left then all the way to the right—with each rotation.

After a few cycles of moving high and low, sliding left then right, Marie looked at me with sheer terror in her eyes. Her arms were outstretched, her knuckles bone white, as she gripped the bar attached to the wall in front of us. The door to the cab was open, and I could see the blacktop below us as I came crashing into her.

The green monster threw us back into the air and Marie slid to the safety of my side of the cab. As we seesawed back toward the ground, I tried with all my might not to crash into her, but I wasn't strong enough. *I'm sorry, I'm sorry, I'm sorry.* I couldn't control my body. I couldn't keep it from flying across the cab and pushing Marie toward certain death. Every time I came toward her, the look on her face begged me to stay on my side. And each time, I failed. I felt like I was being bad, doing something wrong. I was messing up again. I was out of control and Marie was about to die because of it. *I'm sorry, I'm sorry, I'm sorry.*

I don't know how many times this happened before someone realized the door to our cab was open and the ride was stopped. After safely exiting the cab, we headed toward the adults we knew who were running the ring toss game. With my arm outstretched and finger pointing toward the ride, I moved my lips to tell the story, but no sound came out. I kept gasping, trying to speak, but my voice was gone. It wouldn't work. I still didn't have control of my body.

We're complex beings influenced by many things including genetics, culture, circumstance, and our past experiences. My bed-wetting and the trauma of not being able to stop my body from slamming into Marie on that ride could have taught me that I can't control everything about my body, no matter how hard I try. Instead, they contributed to my drive to control everything possible—especially my body.

I turned to controlling my body weight when I was over-whelmed by things I cared about but couldn't control, like the way people perceived me, who asked me out, or my sibling being bullied. I was easily overwhelmed by emotion and took refuge in my efforts to control my eating or exercising. This quickly backfired when my strict dieting led to binging, then the physical discomfort of feeling overly full—combined with the panic about eating so many calories—led to purging by vomiting or overexercising. Thus began a vicious cycle and, ultimately, a habit of starving, binging, and purging.

Long after I loosened the reins on my eating and body weight—never really letting go—the propensity to try to control circumstances and people continued. It manifested in criticism or attempts to manipulate behavior in my relationships with loved ones.

When life circumstances were beyond my control—a pre-mature baby, an autism diagnosis for my child, a divorce—the weight loss slowly creeped up on me. While I was no longer consciously driven by losing weight, I restricted my eating, ignored meals, and frantically exercised. When the weight fell off, I noticed it, felt proud, then told concerned family and friends that I wasn't dieting. I wasn't. But my death grip on having some semblance of control in my life made it impossible for me to allow gaining any of the weight back.

In *A New Earth*, Eckhart Tolle suggests that if we can surrender to the life truths of uncertainty and impermanence, we'll experience less suffering. Surrendering to uncertainty is the opposite of controlling. It's accepting that we really don't have control over much in this life. We can plan, worry, project, prognosticate, but there's little we can know with absolute certainty.

Impermanence is a blessing and a curse. The bad times don't last forever. The good times don't last forever. There's absolutely no way to change this fact, and the more I embrace impermanence, the less stress I feel. When something's going well, I remind myself that it will pass, which helps me stay in the moment and be grateful. When I'm in a life storm, I'm comforted that it will pass. I can look back at many examples of this over the course of my life.

When my eating disorder started in my early teens, I didn't have the perspective or life experience to accept or even understand the truths of uncertainty and impermanence. Today, I find these truths equally freeing and challenging. There are still situations I want to control, fix, change, alter, or manipulate. My aging face and body sometimes taunt me and cause a shame storm that leads to planning a list of things I'll do and won't do over the next thirty days to reverse the effects of aging on my body and mind. The difference now is that I eventually recognize this compulsion for what it is—a bid to play a losing game. Uncertainty abounds and nothing lasts. And that's a gift.

Control is an illusion. We don't have the ability to completely control anything for a sustained period of time. What we do have is the power to make choices in each and every moment that may move things in the direction of our goals. And when things take a turn, we have the ability to accept this uncertainty, remember that it won't last, take a deep breath, and make a choice.

Chapter 9
Comparison

Alayna

On our way to Six Flags Saint Louis the summer before fourth grade, my best friend Emily and I were giddy in the backseat of her mom's red minivan. Six Flags is an amusement park, and we were roller coaster connoisseurs. We probably went every other weekend. We would ride every single ride we could in those few hours, go to Subway for lunch, and then fall asleep on the ride home. Six Flags with Emily was always one of my favorite ways to spend my summer weekends, so why was I comparing my fourth-grade body to hers?

In the backseat of the minivan, Kesha was playing on the radio, and we were dancing and singing, but I was holding my thighs. I got so frustrated because when I looked down at my lap, my legs were touching. My first reaction was to cover them as much as I could with my hands. I couldn't relax. When I looked over at Emily to see if her legs did the same thing, all I could see was that my legs were ten times bigger. It's true, Emily and I have always had very different body types. She's tall and lean with long legs, while I'm short with a muscular build. But I didn't understand why it had to be that way. I was jealous that she could relax and dance to Kesha while I had to keep a secret and sit uncomfortably. My secret was that I wanted to look like her.

My big secret was never exclusive to Emily, though. As I grew up, the secret applied to more and more girls and women. Most of them were my closest friends. My secret made it hard to feel completely happy for their accomplishments. I loved them deeply and fully, but this thought was always in the back of my head: *If I could just look like her, I'd be happy.* Jealousy ate me alive for the majority of my preteen and teenage years.

Since I isolated myself during the worst part of my eating disorder, the only women I could compare myself to were virtual women. I look back at the way I used to scroll through "What I Eat in a Day" YouTube videos, Pinterest diets, models' Instagram profiles, and more, for hours each day. It honestly felt safe to me because it kept me from thinking about my own body and from looking at myself. That is, until I'd get up to go to the bathroom and walk past my mirror. Then all those women I'd seen online sat on a pedestal in my head. Again, my secret would resurface. *Wow, they must be working harder than me—I need to go harder on my run tomorrow.*

My perspective on comparison has changed drastically within the past year. I'm still a teenager, and I still get very jealous of other girls, but I have a belief that I didn't have two years ago. I believe that if two people ate the same foods their entire lives and exercised the same amount and at the same times, they'd still look drastically different. And this isn't just a belief I tell myself to make me feel better. It's the cold, hard truth that we must accept. If Emily and I eat the same and workout the same every day for the rest of our lives, we will still *never* look the same. Everyone needs different types and quantities of food.

The only way to crawl out of the hole of comparison is to accept these facts. I still haven't fully accepted my body for the way it is, but I'm getting there. Because I know that I have a body that no one else on the entire planet has. Nobody knows exactly what I need, and I don't know exactly what other people need. Accepting where you are can be intense, but it allows for growth.

Comparison

Melissa

My daughter Erin was eight years old when she moved to a more competitive level of gymnastics. Parents were discouraged from watching practice, but we were allowed to observe the last fifteen minutes from the balcony. On one occasion, I saw two things from that balcony that made me nervous—and they had nothing to do with calisthenics.

The girls were moving from the beam area to the vault area and were told to line up. Erin ran over to get in line, and another little girl tried to get in front of her. Erin was very assertive in holding her ground. There was turning and nudging and stepping, along with a few words exchanged. I was mortified. Erin wasn't yielding to the other girl. She was standing her ground! This made me extremely uncomfortable as I sat among the other parents and hoped they wouldn't notice. I thought Erin should be polite and not make a scene. (Remember, don't make anyone uncomfortable!) The entire incident lasted about twenty seconds.

The second thing occurred moments later as the places in line were forgotten and the boredom of waiting for their turn set in. The girls started comparing their bellies. It was very obvious from up above what was happening. They were turning to the side and running their hands from their rib cage down their bellies. There was a lot of pointing at each other's bellies, more rubbing, some talking, and even giggling. I felt sick.

"Mama, is my belly fat?" Erin asked about halfway through the drive home.

"It's not fat, Punkie, your body is just right."

"My stomach sticks out farther than the other girls', and somebody said I'm fat."

"Erin, you are NOT fat. Your belly is supposed to look like that," I pleaded. *Please believe me, please believe me.* Erin really wasn't fat or even a little overweight. Her weight and height percentiles were always healthy and proportional at her annual pediatrician visit.

I was always worried that my eating disorder and body image issues would transfer to Erin, so I wanted to say all the right things. I now realize my response could have been better. Shannon, the dietitian who treated Alayna, and whom I saw for several years in my thirties, challenged my thinking around how best to respond when our kids ask if they're fat. Rather than responding the way I did to Erin, she offered that this could be an opening to an age-appropriate dialogue about diet culture.

My effusive response carried the energy of reassuring Erin that she was not *bad*, implying that being fat would be bad. This isn't helpful for any six-year-old. They don't understand the complexity of body composition, and what she was really asking me was whether or not there was something wrong with her. Shannon's message was that this situation could have been an opportunity to explain that our body size doesn't make us good or bad. I could have asked her what she thought it meant to be fat. I could have explained that fat is part of everyone's body and we all need it in order to survive.

This angst to assure her she was normal reinforced the concept of normal as it relates to body shape and size. There isn't really a normal. No two bodies are alike. There's such as a thing as overweight and underweight, but even that is all relative to a plot point determined by some aggregated data used to define normal body weight. And yet, we know that two young women who are the same height and weight could look very different from one another, despite having the same numbers.

According to the *New York Times* article "The Trouble with Growth Charts," the CDC released the first growth chart in 1977. In 2000, it was updated to be more nationally representative. In 2006, the World Health Organization came out with their own chart. The growth chart is the main event of every well-child visit from birth until the child graduates from pediatrics, and it has trained parents to judge the health and wellbeing of their child by comparing them to other kids.

Parents are given percentiles to describe and evaluate their child's growth. If the child is in the seventieth percentile for height, then they're taller than 70 percent of kids their age. A fiftieth percentile reading for weight would mean half the kids weigh more than that child and half the kids weigh less than that child. Purely comparison.

Of course, the metrics related to body size and shape can be meaningful and helpful given the proper context. It's the misapplication of these metrics as an indicator of one's self-worth or value that's problematic.

Comparison and judgment are intertwined. Byron Katie says, "We are humans and we judge. That's what we do."

When I first heard her say this in a recorded session where she was demonstrating how to do "The Work," I yelled, "YES!" We often admonish ourselves and others for judging, but I agree with Katie that it's human nature. Telling ourselves not to judge is futile. It only serves to make us feel guilty or shift to blaming the person we're judging for being so obviously wrong that it's not really a judgment, it's just truth. Being mindful of our judgments and applying deep questioning is helpful in managing stress and in taming the comparison that feeds an eating disorder. Here's an example.

She has really gotten in shape! Look at those abs. I need to step up my game. The twenty-three-year-old I was admiring told me she was participating in exercise challenges issued by someone she follows on Instagram.

Okay. I was thirty years older than this woman, and I was comparing our bodies and feeling motivated to do better. There's so much ridiculousness in this scenario. In addition to being thirty years older, my foot was in a hard cast from over-exercising. What was most ridiculous, and quite sad, was that I experienced the anxiety I get when I feel like I'm not good enough. Once again, I was measuring my self-worth based on how my body compared to an unrealistic standard. In this case, the body of a twenty-three-year-old.

Deep Questioning:

Is it true that I need to do better—more exercise—because my body doesn't compare well to this twenty-three-year-old? I'm fifty-three years old and the amount and type of exercise my body needs, and the way it will respond to that exercise, is going to be different from someone so much younger than me.

Is it really true that if I worked out harder, my body could look like hers? I guess it's possible, but it would take a very long time, and I do know that the bodies of two people of the same height, weight, and age, won't look exactly the same even if they eat and exercise exactly the same.

How does it make me feel when I think this way? I slip back into feeling unworthy and unlovable. I feel out of control and anxious about how much work I need to do, and what food I need to cut out to look that way. I feel awful when I think this way.

Who would I be if I didn't have this thought? Huh. I don't know. Definitely less anxious. Probably more content with myself and my circumstances. Not having thoughts of unworthiness based on how my body compares to others sounds like heaven. Certainly worth practicing.

Is this the best way for me to spend my energy and my precious time? Dear God, no. I barely know how to use Instagram much less figure out how to find the exercise people and keep up with their challenges! I want to write books, read books, and be around people who make me smarter and who are fun. I also want to be a fun person myself. It's not fun to be the one at the table who doesn't eat or the one who skips the party to exercise.

While I just did this exercise now, reflecting on what happened a year ago, I swear I can slip into those feelings like it was yesterday. It may seem elementary to go through the questioning process, but it really works. I do it all the time now. It's especially good to write it down, but even just going through it quickly in my head helps me course-correct when I'm starting to spiral downward.

Chapter 10
Glamorizing Being Sick

Alayna

Perhaps the most confusing part of my eating disorder was the fact that at my sickest, I accomplished quite a bit. I'll try to explain this in a way that makes sense. At my lowest weight and sickest physical state, I was at a turning point in my eating disorder and beginning to make improvements mentally. But my brain will sometimes tell me that those improvements and accomplishments correlate with my sickness. For example, at my lowest weight, I went to State for cross-country, my classmates nominated me for homecoming court, I started a yoga club at school, and I was making more friends.

It sounds like I can attribute my most proud moments to my weight, right? Wrong. These things happened at a time when I was fighting to get my life back. Some of these accomplishments are the very reasons I chose to recover; they gave me a glimpse of what I could have and who I could be without an eating disorder. I used to call it luck that the stars aligned for me when I needed them to. But if you ask me now, I'll tell you that everything started coming together for me because of the hard work my family and I put into my recovery—which is easier said than done.

Some people eat their Oreos by taking the top cookie off and separating the icing from the cookies. I think the Oreo is much better as a whole (especially if you dip it in milk), but that's just my opinion. In my eating disorder, I'd trained my body and my mind to work separately. They no longer listened to each other or worked together. My body was like the icing on an Oreo; my mind the cookies. I'd taken them apart completely. In fact, they were working against one another. And for this reason, recovery didn't make any sense to me. I'd often scream at my parents saying, "How am I supposed to eat when I'm not even hungry?! Aren't I supposed to listen to my body?!" That, my friends, is the catch. I had to re-learn hunger and fullness. And the only way to get those cues back was to reconnect my body and my mind.

I wasn't myself when I was anorexic. I don't even remember several significant stories from that period of sickness. The first time I realized I didn't remember things was when my mom told me I bent a metal fork. She and I were in our kitchen, sitting on the barstools a few months post-recovery. We were reminiscing on how far I'd come, and she said, "You've come a long way since bending that fork!" She smiled and laughed, but I tilted my head and scrunched my eyebrows in confusion.

"What are you talking about?" I asked.

My mom then opened our silverware drawer, reached into the back, and pulled out a metal fork. It was noticeably bent. She explained, "One night at dinner you were so mad at us for making you eat that you bent this fork with your bare hands." That day, I learned that I'd blocked out several other moments. To me, that's proof that my brain wasn't working right.

I'm an extreme yoga enthusiast because it did just the perfect job for me: put me back in one piece. Yoga was something every therapist recommended for me because it's a stress reliever. But I didn't expect it to reconstruct my mind the way it did. I often learned more about myself from yoga than I did from therapy. My yoga mat became my safe place.

One time, I entered the dimly lit therapy room for my session in a sad mood. I don't remember what I was sad about, but I remember feeling like I was stuck in the sad and would be there forever. Kari, my therapist, greeted me with her warm smile as I took a seat on the beige couch. That couch swallowed me every time. Something about that entire room made me feel like I was being hugged. The kind of hug from a person much larger than me, where I could feel 100 percent protected. That day, as soon as I sat on the couch, the comfort made me cry. I didn't cry in therapy often, so Kari understood that I needed something different that day. She pulled out a book from the shelf next to her and said, "We're gonna do a guided meditation."

Kari proceeded to lead me through some breath work at first, and I soon fell into the trance of meditation.

"Fill your belly with air like a balloon."

This was freedom for me, as I was always subconsciously sucking in my tummy, so it would look empty.

"Now, imagine that a magic carpet arrives. It can be whatever you want it to be. This carpet is going to take you to your special place."

I thought of my baby-blue yoga mat. It floated like the magic carpet in *Aladdin*, and it even had a personality. My baby-blue yoga mat was from Dollar General, but I wouldn't sell it for a million dollars. In my head, that mat took me on a ride through clouds. It made turns through the air and moved in waves like a roller coaster. I wasn't on Kari's couch anymore; I was going to my safe place. I was going to reconnect my body with my mind. My mat dropped me off in a forest, the kind with birch trees with thin, white trunks. I walked around like I was the main character in a movie.

Kari's voice was still there and she said, "Now, imagine that there's a door with a golden doorknob."

A door appeared in front of me with a knob so shiny it made me squint. I opened it, walked inside slowly, and behind that door was my safe place. To my surprise, my imagination was so vast that it made sure to include all my favorite people and things in my life. There were white, fluffy rugs, flickering candles, plants, and birds. Even my dog and my family were there. But they weren't just there, they were dancing, motioning me to join them. And I did.

I left therapy with my head high and shoulders back that day. I found my happy place. The state of being present in my body and my mind simultaneously. I include this story about a simple therapy visit because Kari gave me a tool to recover that day: meditation. She gave me recovery tools every visit, like journaling, talking, listening to music, etc., but yoga and meditation were the ones I decided to pursue most often. Before I knew it, I was meditating or doing yoga (or both) every night before bed.

People who work hard get things thrown in their faces 24/7. I picture God laughing at people when they think they've finally got their shit together. He says in a mocking tone, "Oh, just you wait!" And next thing you know, *SPLAT!* That person falls face first in a pile of shit. That's how I felt just about every other day in recovery, and I still fall face-first in a metaphorical pile of shit more times than I can count.

The yoga and meditation made me think so clearly in the moment, but as soon as I'd finish, I'd get eating-disorder messages thrown at my face right and left. For example, every time I'd get on social media, countless videos and posts with big words and perfect models would say "What I Eat in a Day." Of course, how could I resist the shiny messages, the flawless abs, the toned bodies, and the *food*?! Oh my gosh, the pictures of food. I could watch YouTube videos of perfect girls eating for hours on end. It was almost like I was eating with them, except I was starving. My mouth watered at the sight of celery. Raw spinach seemed like a strawberry cheesecake. I'd watch the "What I Eat in a Day" videos only to compare myself to the women on the internet. Most of them were models, and if they weren't models, they were fitness gurus. These were my idols. They had it all. They glamorized undereating. They glamorized being thin. They glamorized being sick. So I did, too.

Any of my close friends can tell you that looking at old pictures of myself when I was sick is a huge no-no. There's still a part of my brain that thinks I was happy when I was sick. I mean, I'm smiling in those old pictures. But I have to constantly remind myself and let others remind me that I was depressed. I wasn't living. I was dying.

Glamorizing Being Sick

Melissa

Their skeletal figures were swallowed by bluish-green scrubs. A yellowish tube was taped to their faces, ran down their sides, and looped up to a bag of tan liquid that hung on the pole they pushed down the hallway to group therapy. *Those are the good girls. They're stronger, more disciplined, more perfect.*

The cheerleader was darling. She had an athletic figure and no fat on her body. In group therapy, she told us she jumped in the pool at dawn every morning before school to swim laps. She was a straight-A student, better than me in every way. *I'll start running every day.*

In that first hospital stay at sixteen, I idolized the anorexic girls and felt shame for being bulimic. I saw anorexia as the pinnacle of control and bulimia its opposite. I was so very wrong.

In my thirties after having two children, I struggled with anorexia and understood that I had no more control over the compulsion to restrict than I did over the compulsion to binge. I did, however, get more attention when I was underweight. Family expressed concern that I was going down a bad path. Friends asked me how I lost all that weight. They wanted to know the secret.

"I wish I could have just a little bit of anorexia." I've heard this countless times as a response to my sharing that I've struggled with eating disorders. Like the people that wanted just a little bit of anorexia, I held on to the story that thin is good, restricting is strength, and thin and sick is better than fat.

This was my excuse for not moving forward with my life. At the same time, it opened doors that brought me happiness. When I entered the hospital, I found people like me and made real connections that I struggled to find outside of therapy. These connections, some friendships that still exist today, were with people of a variety of ages and from many walks of life.

I began to see myself differently, as someone who was lovable. I also saw there was a big world outside of my hometown and my Catholic school, and that people in this world saw me differently than I did. They thought I was kind, fun, smart, worthy, and someone with a lot of potential. The eating disorder became my identity and my entry to this world where compassion was the language, and I was understood.

It's not uncommon for patients to be reluctant or fearful of leaving an inpatient program, even as they spend every day of treatment longing for the day they're free of it. The comfort of a controlled treatment environment and the transference of responsibility for your life and health to a team of experts lightens the load, so you can focus on what underlies your illness and re-enter the world better equipped to cope. My insurance ran out after twenty-eight days and, fortunately, that coincided with my being as prepared as possible to face my life.

As I prepared to return to school after a month away, I was told that no one knew where I'd been and that I shouldn't tell anyone. I was in the hallway walking to my first class when a girl named Cathy came up to me and said, "Where were you? I heard you were in the hospital for bulimia." I was stunned.

I didn't know what to say. I just shook my head and walked away. Eventually, I accepted the shame of this disease and wore it like a chain with a medallion that lay on my chest. It had sharp edges and poked my heart every time I moved.

The only place that felt comfortable to me, the only place that felt like home, was when I was surrounded by others in treatment. This was usually at a group therapy session. In an ironic twist, this sense of belonging may have fueled my eating disorder. These were my people and what we most had in common was that we were sick.

As I continued through high school, still holding onto my eating disorder, I spent a summer in an intensive outpatient program. The treatment team began to talk to me about my risk for becoming "chronic." I was close to the point of no return, and if I didn't start to take this more seriously, I'd have an eating disorder for the rest of my life. There was a pregnant woman in the program that summer and meeting her was a pivotal point in my recovery. I knew I didn't want to still be doing this as a mother.

There was no single moment for me when my eating disorder behavior switched off. It was more like a gradual fizzle with intermittent bursting bubbles along the way, but the prospect of being chronic was the beginning of the end. It was a crack in the tunnel I was living in, through which a light shined, an invitation to an alternative existence.

Eventually, that crack was the size of a sunroof, and then the tunnel became a convertible. Now, the tunnel is just a pile of rocks that I visit every once in a while. I do seem to carry a small stone from its structure wherever I go. Sure, I set it down sometimes because I get busy with the fullness of my life. But I always know where it is, and sometimes it leads me back to the pile of rocks, the old tunnel, where I'm forced to make a choice. Either get back to living and take action to mitigate the overwhelm, or face the dark, cold, and deadly tunnel of an eating disorder.

Getting overwhelmed typically trips the trigger of compulsion to restrict what I eat or to exercise as a form of purging. I have many tools now that I choose as an alternative to these unhealthy behaviors, but there have been times of extreme and prolonged stress when an escape to the structure and embrace of an inpatient treatment program sounded nice.

I'm still in touch with several women with whom I was in treatment. Two of them are among my best friends. One of the women we were in the hospital with has been in and out of treatment facilities for years. A few days after hearing the heartbreaking news she was in treatment again, I happened to be in the midst of what one might call an overwhelm storm. I thought about her and felt envious that her life had narrowed to the tunnel of her eating disorder, to the point that she needed inpatient treatment. I wanted to not care about so many things, to narrow my own focus to being thin. I wanted to escape. I also wanted people to see how much I was hurting or how much they were hurting me. I couldn't adequately express it, but if I was sickly, they'd realize how bad it really was. Fortunately, the security and comfort that being in a treatment program brought wasn't worth the price of admission for me—being sick.

It's easy to look at the altered, filtered, and color-corrected images of women on social media, in magazines, and on the big screen and think you're falling behind—that they're doing life better than you, that they're more perfect than you. Setting aside the fact that most of those images are altered in some way, the sad truth is that most of the people who meet the cultural ideals of a perfect body are miserable. They've given up part of themselves to chase this slippery prize. Rather than spending their energy on finding or pursuing their purpose, they're stuck in the bottomless pit of chasing the perfect body. And, devastatingly, some of them have made themselves seriously ill in this pursuit.

There's nothing glamorous about sickness of any kind. There's nothing beautiful about giving away pieces of yourself and years of your life so someone will find you worthy of a relationship, a job, a "like," or anything. Acceptance from others is fleeting, especially in the world of social media.

The support of others who also struggle with body image and an eating disorder is priceless, but the illness isn't what truly connects us. It's our struggle to navigate life as sensitive, empathic women who were taught their worth came from pleasing and achieving. It's the uncertainty of how to live meaningfully in a world filled with pain and fear. It's our desire to be happy people despite all of that, while also contributing to healing the world. There's nothing glamorous about this work we support one another through. But it *is* beautiful.

Chapter 11
Healthy Addictions

Alayna

We're all prone to making decisions aligned with old habits, even if we've broken those habits. I'm prone to addiction, and I'm prone to taking things to an extreme. I often think of my eating disorder as the way in which I manifested all my emotions and stress: my outlet. So, take away the eating disorder and I'm likely to want to find a new outlet. Well, what's wrong with running being my outlet? Or painting? Or studying? Or going out? I'm prone to becoming addicted to anything.

One of the hardest parts of overcoming my eating disorder was recognizing that I was unhealthy. I mean, all I was doing was exercising and eating only healthy foods, after all—isn't that healthy? But I didn't even have a definition of healthy. If I think back, the way I viewed healthy was: anything that's associated with weight loss and/or looking "better."

Now my definition is: balance.

Sometimes a greasy cheeseburger is healthy for me, according to my new definition. Sometimes a salad is what I crave, so sometimes that's healthy for me. Whatever serves my emotional, physical, and spiritual well-being is considered healthy to me.

Exercise is a tricky addiction for me. I've always loved fitness and exercise, but I got addicted to it, and it made me unhealthy. But that doesn't mean I can't participate in it anymore. It simply means I need to be constantly aware of the "why?" behind my exercise.

During the beginning stages of recovery, my dietitian drastically limited my exercise. I went from running miles, doing yoga, and high intensity workouts every day to just walking or stretching. When Shannon told me my new parameters, I looked at her like she was an alien. Excessive exercise was the last outlet I had to let go of, my final log that kept me afloat in the river of anxiety. I looked to my mom for some help, but by then, she knew that following Shannon's orders was the way to get me healthy. And she was right. I had to learn to be okay with not exercising intensely to truly appreciate exercise.

Today, fitness is always present in my life, and I always want it to be. I see fitness as the best way to celebrate what my body can do, not what it can look like. I know what it's like to not be able to exercise, so I'm aware of how important movement is for my mental health. I'm not going to sit here and say that I have a perfect relationship with exercise, because I don't. Some days I still obsess over the calories listed on my Apple Watch that shows how much I burned during exercise (which, by the way, indicates nothing about the quality of *any* exercise routines). I love to push myself to new limits, but I have to constantly fight the urge to make fitness my only priority in life.

I recognized that I was still obsessing over exercise during the winter of 2020. I was a senior in high school and was on the cross-country team when my right hip started giving me trouble. I ignored it because there's no way I could imagine giving up running. However, my first 5K race of my senior year was a whole four minutes slower than my personal best the previous year. Immediately, I blamed it on all the weight that I'd gained in recovery. But when my teammates and parents told me that I was limping during the race, I was shocked. I was subconsciously pushing myself too hard and forgetting the pain. Soon enough the pain got too bad for me to walk. My hip felt like it could snap at any second, so I walked around like a seventy-year-old, careful to keep my body together.

When I was told that I'd need surgery over Christmas, I broke down. That meant months of no intense exercise and months of slow recovery. During those long months, I noticed just how much I needed exercise for my mental well-being. I was ten times more crabby because I had so much built-up energy I couldn't release. It was a perfect time to reflect on whether I had a healthy relationship with exercise or if it still needed some work. I decided that I still relied on fitness a little too much, and that I'd sucked the fun out of exercise.

Today, I switch up my workouts to keep the fun present, although it's a constant battle in my head. I'm back to running, and I picked up some weight lifting. I feel stronger than I ever have, and I'm proud of it. Sometimes people ask me if I'm afraid to get too "manly" from all the lifting I do. I just laugh and give them a sympathetic smile.

Fitness has more meaning to me now than it ever has. And yes, I sometimes get scared that I'll fall back into the rabbit hole of addiction, but I know better. If I dip my toe into the water of overexercising, I call it out. I tell someone out loud, "Hey, I think I'm overdoing my exercise, and I know it can get unhealthy."

Just the act saying it out loud overrides any obsessive thoughts. I know what life is like without addiction, and I don't ever want to go back to the obsessive life I used to live.

Healthy Addictions

Melissa

In 2020, there was a stay-at-home order in Saint Louis City due to the COVID-19 pandemic. It lasted for sixty-two days. I decided to work out every day until the stay-at-home order was lifted. I posted about my goal and workout streak on Facebook and encouraged others to join with the hashtags #InHonorOf-ThoseWhoAreSick and #InGratitudeForMyHealth. There were several Facebook friends who joined my effort and many dozens who cheered us on.

While I've always been an exerciser, I haven't worked out seven days a week since I was in the throes of an eating disorder, and that was decades ago. At age fifty-one, it seemed like a safe pursuit, and I was mindful that it was for a limited time-frame. Oh, but exercise is tricky. It feels great to me, changes the shape of my body over time, and helps me sleep better at night. During the pandemic, there was the added bonus of giving me space from my family.

I lived with my kids and my partner, and he and I walked at least two miles together daily, usually four, but I didn't count that as my exercise. I think that when I started the exercise streak, I intended for those walks to count. But subtly, almost imperceptibly, rules began to pop up. The only exercise that counted was the morning workout, which consisted of either a ride on the Peloton, a minimum of thirty minutes on the Nordic-Trak, or a three-to-four-mile run. Then, I started adding "mat work" like abdominal exercises and lifting weights. Before I knew it, I was walking four to six miles a day on top of my morning workouts. I LOVED it. And I was exhausted.

It became evident after the second week that this would be impossible for me to keep up if I was going into the office each day. I needed more sleep than what would be required if I were to do a daily workout "that counted," get ready for work, and be at work on time. I could do it for a couple of days, but by the third day, I'd be too tired to get up at 5:00 a.m. When working from home, I could push it to a 7:00 a.m. workout and just not shower before walking upstairs to my 8:30 a.m. meeting. I started to have anxiety about what I'd do when I had to go back to the office.

This is what happens to me with exercise. I start thinking ahead and worrying about how I'll keep it going. When I'm in the vortex of exercise addiction, and I know I have upcoming travel, I start planning how I'll get in my exercise. Each run has to be as fast as the last run, if not just a little faster. Doing a twenty-minute bike ride isn't enough if I'd deemed thirty minutes a "real" workout. Skipping the mat work stopped being an option.

Running has always been my Achilles' heel, so to speak. When I was ten years old, I started getting up in the morning before school and running around the block. There's no exercise that makes me feel better than running. I get into a zone, and it's akin to meditation for me. During the stay-at-home order, I started running more. I was still mixing it with the bike and the NordicTrak, but running started to overtake the other exercises.

About forty days into the stay-at-home order, my right foot started hurting at the ball of my foot just south of my big toe. I'd felt that pain before when I wore heels for too long, but what started as a nagging pain when I ran really started to hurt. I didn't stop running. I noticed that it only hurt when I started running, and then it sort of went away. It actually became numb after about a quarter-mile. Instead of accepting that this was probably not a good sign medically, I was thrilled that I'd found the trick to keep running. No matter how badly it hurt at first, it would eventually go numb, and I could get my four miles in! Don't worry; I'm shaking my head with you.

The pain started to show up when I was taking walks with my partner. That worried me because those walks were golden for our relationship. We got to step away from the crazy work-loads, worry over the kids and the news, and simply enjoy the spring weather and one another.

I made it through my sixty-two days, finishing with a 10k run in the rain on the last day. And that was the end of my forty-one-year running career. After four months jockeying between an orthopedic boot and a hard cast, I was diagnosed with necrosis of the sesamoid bone. Necrosis means death. I had literally run that bone to death and had to have it surgically removed.

"Healthy" addictions are tricky. Even when we're aware of our susceptibility to becoming addicted, it's so easy to tell ourselves that what we're doing is healthy. It's also easy to seek and receive reinforcement for what we're doing.

I stopped eating meat in 2008 after watching a documentary about the food production process in the United States, which included many disturbing visuals of how animals are treated in that process. In 2011, I tried a vegan diet after watching a film that shared information and testimonies about plant-based diets aiding in the control and prevention of chronic diseases such as diabetes and cancer. I'm not recommending either film so I'm not naming them, especially if you're someone who struggles with an eating disorder or tends to create rules around food. Watching these films and seeing these visuals only served to fuel my restrictive tendencies, and they all but destroyed my ability to enjoy many foods I really loved and that contain nutritional value.

I convinced myself that my choice to eat a plant-based diet was based solely on the treatment of animals in the food production process. I'd researched a few more videos and found arguments that dairy cows and hens are also treated poorly, so no eggs, milk, or cheese either. I was kidding myself. What started as an ethical reason for those restrictions quickly shifted when I saw the slimming effects on my body. The problem was that I was hungry all the time. You can only eat so many nuts and seeds, especially when you're exercising, and I've always been terrible at meal planning. The only way to eat a plant-based diet and get the right amount of nutrition is to plan your meals *and snacks*. Oh, and go grocery shopping. And at fifty-three, I'm still afraid of the grocery store—so much food—so that was a problem.

I eventually went back to eating meat and dairy. It was so freeing to walk into a sandwich shop and realize that I could choose from anything on the menu! This also applied to Italian restaurants and pizza parlors.

Special diets are challenging for people with eating disorders or those tendencies, but they're sometimes necessary for health reasons. The medical excuse to restrict makes it easy to start restricting things that aren't medically necessary to avoid, and it can be a slippery slope.

In a stroke of irony, I now have difficulty digesting dairy. Now, while I still eat mostly plant-based foods, if I want sushi, I eat it. If I want steak, I have some. It's even more freeing to know that I can eat what's comfortable for me to digest and what I like. Rule-free.

My mother used to say, "MODERATION, Melissa." I hated that word. I didn't do it well. I still don't sometimes, depending on how chaotic life feels. Here are a few things I do to keep myself from getting sucked into my "healthy" addictions.

I move every day, even if it's just to walk the dog.

I meditate. This has helped with body awareness, which makes it easier for me to notice when my body has had enough of or needs something.

I don't label my eating. No labels. No rules.

Because cardiovascular exercise helps me sleep better at night, I'm now doing ten-minute rides on the Peloton if that's all I can fit in.

It's a new paradigm for me to see exercise as a way to nurture my body rather than wanting to be thinner and punishing myself for overeating.

Chapter 12
Triggers

Alayna

I have a hard time hearing the word *trigger*. It builds up flames in my body. Why? Well, simply put, there's nothing quite like trying to recover from a life-threatening illness, while the rest of the world is promoting everything that goes against your recovery, a.k.a. triggers. In my experience, anytime someone says or does something triggering, I immediately assume they're against me.

One day in an appointment with my dietitian, I learned that people with eating disorders tend to focus on numbers. The number on the scale, the number of minutes of exercise, and especially the number of calories eaten. After that appointment, I repeated to myself *don't look at the numbers.* I said this in my head over and over again while my mom and I drove to get lunch. When we got in line to order, I looked at the menu. All I saw was: *150 cal., 1500 cal., 325 cal., 750 cal.* The more numbers I saw, the faster my heart started beating. I couldn't think about what I was craving, because what if I was craving the food that was 1,500 calories?

This still happens to me when I order from menus that list calories. The numbers trigger the eating disorder part of my brain. However, I now know that the menu creators aren't making me suffer on purpose. It took me a long time to realize that no one was against me; in fact, I was once like them. I was once ignorant to the world of eating disorders and ignorant to what could trigger people in recovery.

This realization manifested itself in my junior year high school writing class. Through this class, I was able to choose my own topics to write about. It soon became a way for me to forgive those who triggered me and to educate my classmates and teachers on the reality of eating disorders. I wrote an argument paper on why restaurants shouldn't list calories on their menus. It was the best paper I've written to this day.

I used to get triggered in class too often. It could be as simple as my classmate saying "Ugh, I haven't worked out in so long. I need to!" Or, saying right before lunch, "I'm staaarving," or, "I haven't eaten all day." These are things people haven't stopped saying, and probably never will stop saying. But at the time, I immediately resented them for triggering me.

To avoid getting in verbal fights, I'd force myself to leave the class and sit in the bathroom for five minutes. I usually texted my mom too. It got so routine that eventually I'd text my mom "bathroom time," and she knew that meant someone said something triggering. It wasn't an overnight switch that changed my mindset from resentment to acceptance. I had to work at it. And let me tell you, it's not an easy skill to be able to accept and understand someone that's triggering. I like to think, *If I never had an eating disorder, would I say those things, too?* And nine times out of ten, the answer is yes. So, I'm united with the person who triggered me.

Two years later, I'm still hypersensitive to what people say and do regarding food, exercise, and body image. I'll probably always feel anxious when someone says they aren't hungry because I start to feel jealous, but I feel less resentful. They're human and they don't intend to trigger me.

My biggest trigger has always been pictures of myself. Getting "cute pictures" with friends is bound to happen at any occasion. I hate it. But pictures are such a large part of society and belonging, so I put up with them. The reason pictures trigger me is because I used to take pictures of myself in a bra and underwear every morning in my mirror just to make sure I didn't look bigger than yesterday's picture. I still have those photos.

For months during my recovery, when I looked at those photos, I saw a chubby girl. Now when I look at them, all I see is the expression of hopelessness on my face. I shiver when I see them because I remember how I felt in those moments. How blind I was to the damage I was doing. So, when a friend asks me to take a picture, I have a strategy now. I say yes, and I make sure to be doing something in the picture that shows how happy I am. Whether it be hugging my friend, making a silly face, or just smiling as big as I can. That way, when I look at it later, I'll be able to notice the expression of joy on my face. That change alone has made recovery worth it.

Triggers

Melissa

About six months after the surgery to remove the overexercised dead bone in my foot, my daily exercise streak had long passed, and I was back to my ebb and flow of good weeks and bad weeks. I was at my general practitioner's office for a physical. They had a machine that measures a number of factors about body mass, including how much water is in your system at the time. It then gives you a score of red, yellow, or green for each of the factors and compares you to other people of the same age and gender denoted by a percentile.

I happened to be having a really bad day related to body image. My life was a bit of a mess. My job had recently changed due to a merger, I'd ended my four-year relationship and moved out of my partner's house, and my dog had just died. I was sad and scared. The doctor, who knew I had a history of eating disorders, started asking me what I eat every day. Bad move. I reminded her that I eat mostly vegan but don't label myself accordingly because it helps me remain flexible. I reminded her of my history of eating disorders. She then started talking to me about how much protein I should be getting and how much exercise I needed based on recommendations from the American Heart Association. *Oh my God, please shut up.* Then came the report card. The percentiles. The green, yellow, and red indicators of performance level.

My brain was going a mile a minute. I wanted to Google definitions of all the indicators. She started talking through it, and I sat there with my arms crossed, hands squeezing my arms. The more she talked, the harder I squeezed. I wanted to understand all of it. I wanted to know what it meant, but I was afraid of it. I told her the report stressed me out. She tried to encourage me by showing me how good my numbers were, pointing to all the green graphs. *But that one is yellow. How much water am I supposed to have in my body?* When it was finally over and we were moving on to the next topic, she pushed the report toward me and said, "This is your copy."

She changed the subject to my supplements and medications, but I wasn't listening. I was obsessing over the yellow graphs. After about thirty seconds, I interrupted her. Pushing the report back across the table to her, I said, "I don't want this. It's not good for me to have those numbers."

She nodded her head and continued going through the supplements, then interrupted herself to say, "Are you sure? These numbers are really good! Just take it in case you need to be reminded."

We'd already started working on this book, so I texted Alayna and told her what happened. I was so angry. I told her about how I tried to advocate for myself and how the practitioner didn't hear me. The doctor was well-intentioned, but it reminded me how little even some healthcare professionals understand about the triggers for people with eating disorders. The paper sat on the passenger seat of my car for a couple of days before I glanced at it once more and threw it out. It didn't set me back.

Triggers are highly individual. One person can be triggered into unhealthy thoughts or a downward spiral by seeing calories on a menu, while another person can shrug that off. Identifying your triggers is important, so you can have a plan for each of them. For example, I'm triggered when I see my weight on the scale, so I don't have a scale in my home. When I'm at the doctor's office, I turn around when they weigh me and ask them not to say my weight aloud.

Calories on a menu don't bother me, but people talking about the healthiness or unhealthiness of their food or mine, especially while we're eating, is upsetting to me. If this is someone in my family, I address it immediately. Otherwise, I change the subject with the intention of addressing it later if it's someone with whom I'll be eating again.

As important as it is to have a plan for the things that trigger you, it's equally important not to panic when they arise or when a new one appears. Everyone is set off by something. This is where it's really helpful to have a mindfulness practice. If the thought of that is overwhelming, just start listening to your body by focusing on your breath. The next time you start to get angry or stressed out about something (and it's probably best to practice with an issue that's unrelated to eating), ask yourself where you feel that stress or anger in your body. Is it in your throat? Your chest? Your gut? Are your shoulders up by your ears?

Focusing on where you feel the stress building in your body can help quiet the mental chatter. Once you find that tightness in your body, imagine you can direct your breath in and out of that spot. This focus on your breath should calm your nervous system.

For example, if the stress has forced your shoulders to your ears, drop the shoulders and imagine each breath going into the space between your shoulder blades. Then imagine that with each breath, there's a peaceful light glowing in that area. If you have time to stick with this, you can imagine the light spreading throughout your body. By this point, the mental chatter will be very dull, and you can now rationally consider what choice you want to make in response to whatever triggered you.

For the loved ones of people struggling with an eating disorder, there's often great fear that they'll say or do something wrong or triggering. I'm often asked about the best way to talk to a child, sister, or friend with an eating disorder. "I don't want to say the wrong thing," is often conveyed with earnestness, love, and many times, tears. Unfortunately, there's no playbook for this. As I've noted above, well-intentioned health care professionals are often misguided. In fact, it's okay that my doctor triggered me. It was unintentional. The problem was, she didn't hear me either time I told her the report wasn't good for me.

The best advice I can give anyone in this situation is to *listen.* Practice empathy and validate the feelings being expressed. Listen closely and ask a few questions to help further your understanding. If they ask you to stop, don't try to reinforce your position by explaining your intentions. Just let it go. It's okay. This will build trust over time, and it best positions you to remain in a relationship where you're learning from each other.

Part 3: Guideposts

You're allowed to be here fully. Say that out loud: "I'm allowed to be here fully." You won the cosmic lottery, and you're here on this planet. You're allowed to fully be who you are.

When you choose the path of starvation, it isn't only your body that's empty. When you deny your body nourishment through binging and purging, all aspects of your life are out of balance. Your relationships with others suffer, and sometimes the damage is irreparable. More significantly, your connection to your true self, the part of you that clearly sees your gifts and knows how to use them, is broken. But there's a way back.

Most importantly, you need medical attention. Eating disorders are diseases that can kill you. At the very least, they rob you of the beauty of daily life and steal your energy. According to the National Association of Anorexia Nervosa and Associated Disorders (ANAD), anorexia has the highest death rate of any psychiatric illness. Think about that. One is more likely to die from anorexia than major depression. ANAD reports that without treatment, up to 20 percent of people with serious eating disorders die. This rate falls to 2 percent to 3 percent with treatment. ***Get medical help.***

Full: Overcoming Our Eating Disorders to Fully Live

Following are actions that have become handrails for us as we move up and down the staircase of life. We're often able to move along quickly without disruptive thoughts, but when the light dims, or we're tired and start to stumble, we grab onto one or more of these handrails to help us stay on track with our health.

Personal Practices that Can Help

Alayna

Being stuck is a horrible state. I remember getting my foot stuck in the wooden panels at the end of my toddler bed as a child, and I woke up in complete agony at the feeling of being stuck. It's uncomfortable and can lead to uncontrollable panic. You *can* get out. Many of the following guideposts are examples of practical tools to escape your consuming negative thoughts. Your first step, however, is to get up. Stand up. Take a step. Then you've completed the hardest part of escaping from being stuck.

Create

Find a spot, preferably in nature, where you likely won't be disturbed. Mine is a room in my house surrounded by windows through which I can see the trees. Everyone has the ability to create *something*. Maybe it's a painting, a pencil drawing, a poem, a song, a dance, or a continuous squiggly line on a blank piece of paper. Whatever comes effortlessly to you, do it, and do it unapologetically. Maybe you will surprise yourself.

Move

Healthy movement can be a tricky thing for the eating-disordered brain to understand. As humans, we need movement and exercise to keep us mobile and energized. Exhaustion is the opposite of that. Make a list of every type of movement you participate in. Then, mark which types are driven by unhealthy motives. My unhealthy motives were usually things like weight loss, burning calories, or beating myself up. What you're trying to do now is to find the types of movement that will help you escape the negative thoughts in your head. Therefore, by identifying which movements don't serve you in that space, you can begin to focus on those that do serve you.

Yoga is my go-to movement for getting out of my head. Every single time I do yoga, it comes from a place of self-care, not self-degradation. Walking outside is also a healthy escape for me. It's important to note that movement doesn't need to be categorized as a "workout." Rather, movement can be as simple as touching each of your fingertips to your thumb, or patting your head while rubbing your stomach. Your brain will begin to focus on the small task at hand, without creating the stress that an exhausting workout would create. Movement is powerful, but it's not the only way to escape your thoughts, so remember to check in with the interior motives behind your chosen movement.

Journal

In a lifetime fitness class as a freshman in college, I learned that about 100,000 chemical reactions occur in the average brain every second. I also learned that your sleeping brain could power a twenty-five-watt bulb. That's a lot of power and an overwhelming amount of information to sift through. No wonder you feel down in those moments when most of your thoughts are negative. You might be unaware of those thoughts, which is why it's important to acknowledge them sometimes. An easy way to take note of your thoughts is to write them down. Journaling forces you to sort through your thoughts. It doesn't have to look a certain way, which is the beauty of journaling.

Find a notebook or a scrap of paper and write whatever comes to mind. My journal is full of all different styles of writing. Some of my entries are prayers, some are full of cuss words, some are lists, some are sentences. No matter what journaling style speaks to you, I encourage you to write the date of your entry each time you journal. Save your entries, no matter how ridiculous. Then, your future self will be able to look back and be proud of everything you've gone through. If you're not sure what to write, take a look at this simple exercise I've done a few times:

1. Ten things you're grateful for
2. Ten things you look forward to
3. Ten things you want to accomplish
4. Ten things you can improve upon
5. Put your pen, pencil, or marker to a blank page and see which direction your mind wants to wander

Service

You can't help others unless you've helped yourself first. However, sometimes helping others and yourself go hand in hand. On my own recovery journey, I first had to do the work with my therapist and dietitian. But one day, I decided that sharing my struggles with others would be beneficial to me and those I'd share with. That day, I was going on a bike ride with the boy I was dating at the time and his little sister. She was a teenager, a few years younger than me. After our bike ride, she claimed that she felt skinny because she hadn't eaten all day and had just finished a workout. Although she meant it as a casual comment, I couldn't bear the thought of another young girl thinking the way I used to in my eating disorder. I broke down in the parking lot, held onto my bike and sobbed, holding my chest.

That night, I posted this on my snapchat story: "Let me know if anyone would want to be added to a private story where I'll post about my struggles and triumphs in eating disorder recovery." In only one day, one hundred people—all girls that I knew—begged to be added. From that point on, I learned the importance of serving people the way I wanted to be served. I didn't want to stop there, so at my high school, I started a yoga club. I was the "instructor," and we'd do simple yoga and meditation during the school day to relieve stress. About two hundred girls signed up for the yoga club, and even though I've graduated, the school still operates that club.

Service doesn't look the same for everyone, but it always prompts deeper human connection. My service was letting people know they weren't alone, but your service might be something completely different. First, take care of yourself, and when you're ready to dive deeper into recovery, find an area of your life to give back to people. I promise you will be enlightened.

Faith

"When faith is blended with the vibration of thought, the subconscious mind instantly picks up the vibration, translates it into its spiritual equivalent and transmits it to Infinite Intelligence." This is something I learned from the book *Think and Grow Rich* by Napoleon Hill.

I wouldn't have recovered without my faith. It's a simple fact. Growing up in the Catholic church set a strong foundation for my faith, and I'm beyond grateful that I remembered to cling to my faith during my anxiety and depression. Oftentimes, I felt the pressure to be a perfect Catholic, but in the depths of my struggles, I realized that having faith alone was enough. I believe in God, and I believe I went through my eating disorder for a purpose. I believe that God answered my prayers and cries for help. When I lost myself, at least I still had my faith. I encourage you to have faith, whether it be religious or not, because it will give you the purpose you've been searching for.

Personal Practices that Can Help

Melissa

Connect

We're social beings who are sustained by our connections to others. Brené Brown defines connection as the energy that exists between people when they feel seen, heard, and valued, when they can give and receive without judgment, and when they derive sustenance and strength from the relationship.

Isolation, loneliness, and depression are opposites of connection, and when we're in those mindsets, reaching out to someone can feel like moving a mountain. Prepare for those moments by making a list of three to five people you can reach out to when you find yourself spiraling out of control or past that point and swimming in a pool of destructive behavior. There's no guarantee that the first person you call or text will be available. Commit to going through your list until you find someone who has ten minutes to chat.

The people on your list are unlikely to be therapists, and it's not their responsibility to fix you or change your mindset. That's your responsibility. The purpose of this connection is to pull you out of the rut of your current thinking or behavior. My experience is that talking about my issues in those moments with someone other than a therapist only perpetuates unhealthy thinking, giving it a voice. The purpose of this conversation is to change the scenery of my mind and quiet that negative inner voice.

When in the pit of darkness, figuring out what to say can be a barrier to making the call. On the same page that you wrote your list, write an opening line for the discussion, such as, "Hey. I just need to get out of my own head for a while and remember there's a great big world out there. Do you have a few minutes to chat?"

You can follow that by asking a few exploratory questions to get the conversation going, such as: "What's going on in your world? What's your favorite thing to do when life sucks? What makes you laugh the hardest?"

While this may seem like overkill, knowing exactly how to start the conversation will do two things for you: 1) It removes the excuse of not knowing what to say, and 2) it reminds you the discussion needs to center on something other than your issues.

Shifting your attention to other topics or people puts space between an impulse and an action. Sometimes all we need is just a break in the pattern so we can make a different choice.

Give It Away

I once read that if you find yourself feeling desperate for something, reach out and give that very thing to someone else. For example, when you feel like no one understands you, try to understand someone who you find challenging. When you feel like you don't have enough money, leave a tip anyway, even if it's just a nickel. When you're feeling down, look for someone to cheer up.

When I remember to do this, it's always rewarding. And it works! I start feeling better, more abundant, and more connected to others. This also reminds me that what I need to feel better is within *me*. Sometimes the best way to access what's inside of us is to call it out for someone else.

Practice Gratitude

An article titled "Giving Thanks Can Make You Happier," posted by Harvard Health Publishing, says "With gratitude, people acknowledge the goodness in their lives. In the process, people usually recognize that the source of that goodness lies at least partially outside themselves. As a result, being grateful also helps people connect to something larger than themselves as individuals—whether to other people, nature, or a higher power."

In short, gratitude is the secret sauce for happiness. Gratitude has become a hot topic in positive psychology research which studies the strengths, characteristics, and actions that help people and communities thrive. While researchers stop short of saying that gratitude causes happiness, studies consistently show an association between gratitude and happiness.

Gratitude can be applied to both past events and things happening today. Some even give thanks for future things with the intention of manifesting those into their reality. In my experience, the practice of gratitude can't be overdone, and it's extremely effective in those moments when things feel terrible. As with connection, and many of the other guideposts we offer, the practice of gratitude shifts your focus from the pain, fear, and negativity to the larger picture. When we broaden our perspective, there's always something beautiful, even if we have to look far beyond the current situation to find it.

Many people swear by a daily gratitude practice like writing down five things they're grateful for before bed each night, with the goal of the nightly list not being repetitive. This is harder than it sounds, so you find yourself seeking things throughout the day to put on your list. That openness to beauty borders on an expectation of good things happening, which is a fundamental shift from a fearful, negative outlook that's common in periods of depression and in the throes of an eating disorder. It's impossible to be filled with both gratitude and fear at the same moment.

Find a regular gratitude practice that works best for you and remember that it's a great tool to use when you're feeling especially down or desperate. Widening your perspective to see the beauty will bring you back into balance.

Practice Mindfulness

There are two ingredients to mindfulness: 1) embodied awareness, and 2) acceptance. Embodied awareness means that you're paying attention to how the present moment is resonating in your body. Acceptance means that you don't ruminate on or judge what you notice; you just remain open and curious.

When I practice mindfulness, I start by focusing on my breath, then on each of the five senses singularly. Throughout this process, I return to my breath for check-ins and usually find I need to unclench my belly and drop my shoulders.

I'm currently in my home office which doubles as my Zen studio. When I work from home, this is where I work. When I do yoga or meditate, this is my studio. It's helpful to take mindfulness breaks while I'm writing. This is what one looks like for me right now:

- I focus on my body and notice that my abdominal muscles are clenched and my breathing isn't smooth. I take a deep breath and relax my stomach, which helps the air move through my body more deeply. My next breath makes my stomach extend and my lungs fill.
- I notice my legs are crossed. I uncross them and feel my toes touch the carpet. I move my feet back and forth along the carpet and feel the fuzzy texture. My breath comes deeply without even thinking.
- I feel my shoulders drop from my ears. My belly gets bigger with each filling breath. It feels so good.
- I hear the clicking of the keys and feel the pads of my fingertips depress the silicone keyboard cover.
- I notice my hair touching my cheek and see the ends of that lock subtly moving back and forth from the breeze of the ceiling fan.

- I hear the soft piano music coming from the speaker on the table to the left of me.
- I look away from the keyboard to the beautiful painting of lilies in a pond and the sky reflecting off the water.
- I smell the lavender and sage scents coming from the candle on my desk.
- I notice I'm starting to get hungry.
- Out of the corner of my right eye, I see my fluffy, black, Cavapoo puppy napping.

Mindfulness is an active form of meditation. The principles of focused attention and absence of judgment apply to both meditation and mindfulness, but mindfulness is used while performing an act, like walking up the stairs, typing a chapter of a book, or eating your dinner.

I practice both meditation and mindfulness and have found that my nervous system is generally less reactive since I started. My threshold for frustration is higher, and I'm generally more calm. I'm not less sensitive. In fact, I've probably cried more in the past year than in previous years, and I believe that's because I'm not only allowing myself to feel, but I'm actively pursuing discovery of my emotions in any given moment.

While the thought of being more sensitive may sound threatening, those feelings are there, and those bodily sensations are happening whether we focus on them or not. Mindfulness breaks can serve as a pressure release valve, giving us the space to process the little things so that they don't become a major issue or drive us to compulsive, unhealthy behaviors.

Do Body Check-Ins

Body check-ins are like mindfulness snacks for me. I'm working on creating a check-in habit, so I don't get too far into discomfort before I remember to focus on what's happening inside. A check-in is a quick body scan for tension or blockages. The first place I usually find tension is in my belly, with my shoulders being a close second. As I find the tension, I focus on breathing into it. Sometimes I find I'm clenching my jaw. Some people notice clenched fists or sweaty palms. The key here is to recognize that your body is telling you something.

I use body check-ins when I have to make a decision. For example, I'm writing this as the Omicron variant of the Coronavirus is running rampant throughout the country. My sister, Colleen, called me yesterday and offered a gift to my family. She and her husband would like to "sponsor" our New Year's Eve celebration. My little family has had a tough year including major life changes that we didn't see coming, and Colleen and Paul (my brother-in-law) want to help us kiss the year goodbye and usher in the new year with joy.

Colleen offered a few suggestions, not knowing what made the most sense for us with my daughter's health condition and the state of COVID-19 in our town. One of her suggestions was a night in a hotel. I really liked the idea of the kids and me doing something dramatically different than in other years, like staying in a hotel to ring in the new year. I started scrolling online resources for finding a cabin within driving distance of the hospital, so that we could take our dog and have no worries about being around other people.

After ten minutes of research, I noticed I wasn't breathing deeply, my shoulders were at my ears, and my jaw was clenched—the trifecta. I started breathing into my belly until it loosened up and started sticking out with each inhale. My shoulders came down on their own with the first breath. I focused on relaxing my cheeks and letting my jaw feel heavy. Then, there was clarity. Going to a hotel or cabin would make me anxious for a number of reasons. This is directly contrary to the goal of having a joyful celebration. My body was my guide to accepting that this is just not our year to spend the night away on New Year's Eve.

Next, I decided to use my body check-in to consider dinner out on New Year's Eve. I focused on my breath and asked myself if dinner out felt like a safe, enjoyable activity for that night. I imagined us at a busy restaurant—there's no other kind on New Year's Eve—and felt my stomach tighten. Strike two.

Finally, I imagined us at home, eating our favorite foods and desserts from our favorite restaurants, the fire going, the puppy driving us crazy while simultaneously making us coo with adoration, and playing games at the dining room table. Voilà! No tension in the shoulders, no stress. Decision made.

Body check-ins can also be helpful when you're feeling anxious. Ask yourself where you feel the anxiety in your body. Scan your entire body. You will likely find the usual suspects, which for me are stomach, shoulders, and jaw, but you may also find that your toes are curled, or that your crossed legs are pressing tightly against one another rather than resting.

The more you practice mindfulness, the better you will be at body check-ins, and if you develop a habit of body check-ins, mindfulness will become more natural to you.

Be a Lifelong Learner

The single most significant contributor to my freedom from the eating disorder has been my commitment to learning about the many ways people find contentment and peace in their lives. I find comfort in researched-backed methods or information, such as Brené Brown's work on shame, Charles Duhigg's book, *The Power of Habit*, or the skills defined in Marsha Linehan's *Dialectical Behavior Therapy*. For virtually every aspect of personal development, you can find information and methods supported—or challenged—by research.

Don't discount the power of personal stories. Nejwa Zebian's *Welcome Home: A Guide to Building A Home for Your Soul* is a great example of a book crafted from personal experience that helped me understand myself better. *The 5 Love Languages: The Secret to Love that Lasts* by Gary Chapman helped me understand what actions make me feel most loved and the way in which I most often show my love. Glennon Doyle's *Untamed* is an insightful, hilarious, sad, and motivating book on women's issues.

Personal narratives can be more relatable than research, and I often find my way back home to myself by reading a story or blog post by someone who's dealing with something similar. The personal development genre of books, blogs, and videos can be just the hand you need to get back on track or feel reconnected with other humans when you're feeling alone or like there has to be a better way to get through this life.

Ride the Waves

The biggest lesson I've learned in my fifty-three years on this planet is that there's no plateau on which life becomes easy and we experience eternal happiness. The self-help genre is filled with numbered lists promising happiness, greater wealth, and better self-confidence if we just do <newest action list>. The beauty industry perpetually makes us the promise of younger, sexier, more beautiful skin and bodies if we just use <latest product>. The fitness world promises stronger bodies, six-pack abs, and smaller dress sizes if we just do this <list of exercises>.

Greek philosopher Heraclitus is credited with saying, "The only constant is change." My high school English teacher said this repeatedly, and it made my stomach clench every time. How was I supposed to be perfect and in control when things are constantly changing?

Nothing lasts. Nothing. Lasts. The good feelings don't last. The bad feelings don't last. Young, elastic skin doesn't last. Six-pack abs don't last. LIFE doesn't last. We're all on this planet for a limited amount of time. There's beauty in that fact. Reminders of our impermanence can help us define our priorities. Accepting the impermanence of bad times breeds hope and fortitude.

Acknowledging the impermanence of joyful moments can fuel gratitude for what's happening in the present.

These guideposts and the hundreds of books, articles, videos, and podcasts I've consumed haven't kept bad or difficult things from happening in my life. Life will continue to throw us curveballs. Being committed to learning helps us adapt, adjust, and grow from our experiences so that when the bad times come, we can manage them without doing harm to our bodies or our minds. Understanding how others navigate life and find contentment *in a given moment,* can inspire tools to help us find contentment *in a given moment.*

Life offers the full spectrum of events and emotions, from agony to extreme joy. Understanding what helps you manage your feelings as you move back and forth throughout that continuum is the greatest gift you can give yourself. What works for you as a teenager may not work in the context of adulting or parenting. This is why the commitment to learning is lifelong.

Find Your Faith

Religion has been a double-edged sword for me. From birth until my early forties, I participated in various sects of Christianity. I credit my strong faith in love and a higher power to my early religious training. I felt God in that church. I absorbed the energy and love of a community that believed in and strived to catalyze a greater good.

I stepped away from religion when I realized I was dismissing more of the dogma than I embraced. Some teachings and my interpretation of parts of the doctrine were harmful to my self-worth as a young girl, and I've spent a lifetime unwinding the harmful beliefs that I formed as a result.

"Spiritual but not religious" is a mantra that emerged in the early 2000s. This is professed by those who don't subscribe to a formal religion or religious doctrine but for whom it's important to state that faith, or spirituality, is part of their life. I fall in this camp, and my spirituality plays a significant role in my ability to find contentment and peace.

For me, mindfulness and meditation are spiritual practices. I find God there. I feel the angels, get clarity, and feel truth. Meditation is a form of prayer for me. Sometimes I ask questions. Sometimes I praise God, the earth, and the angels, masters, and guides in service to the evolution of my soul. Sometimes I just listen to my crazy brain that never stops talking. All of it feels holy. I feel connected to something, someone, a community of souls, and that's healing for me.

I can also find this feeling in nature. Just looking at the sky reminds me that this universe is so much bigger than me and that I'm supported. Flowers speak to me. Not literally, but their beauty is magical, and I'm reminded that there are so many things in this world that I don't have to control, that I have nothing to do with, and that's helpful when I'm feeling overwhelmed by my current circumstances.

The mind-body-spirit age is upon us. There are many resources and paths to finding what works for you. The most important thing to keep in mind is that there isn't one right way to find it or to express it. We're ever-evolving, and what worked in grade school doesn't always work in high school.

What worked in my thirties didn't work for me in my forties. Now, in my fifties, I'm no more or less "good" because of the way I practice faith than when I was participating in religion. I do know that without my connection to spirit, my life would be so much harder. I know this because there have been periods of my life when I stepped away from spirituality altogether and relied only on my mind and body to get by.

Faith, in whatever form it takes for you, can be a lifeline when the world feels too loud, messy, or unkind. When you're staring down a runway of change, and you feel drained by the road behind you, a spiritual practice can be a source of energy. It can fill you up.

A Letter to the Reader

Alayna

The idea for this book came to fruition because of the countless times I've witnessed girls and women missing out on life because of the way they felt about their bodies. I used to think having a bad body image was a sign of inferiority. Now, I see it as a point of unity. We all struggle with self-acceptance, and yet we hide it to save face.

I'm no different than you. I don't wake up every day with a smile on my face and open my curtains with gratitude for the sunshine. The truth is, I still have bad body image days that compel me to restrict my eating or to hide my body. But, my hope for you and I is bigger than the voice in my head telling me I'm not enough. I don't want to be a mother who thinks she needs to go on a diet before going on a beach vacation. I want to be a badass woman free of restrictions and limitations.

Most of all, I want YOU to be badass and free of limitations. I want YOU to tell the voices in your head to "fuck off" when they tell you you're not enough.

What I want for you won't change anything, I know that. But I need you to know that I'm cheering you on.

Whatever voice you're battling right now, let me be the first to tell it that it's full of shit.

I wrote this for you, to inspire the confidence you've buried deep within your soul. I want you to seek out this confidence, knowing that it will carry you beyond the set of beliefs about yourself that you thought were true.

Then, maybe, hopefully, one day you'll be able to fully live.

Love,

Alayna

A Letter to the Reader

Melissa

You've helped me heal. When I shared with friends that I'd be writing this book with Alayna, a common response was that it would probably be a healing experience for me. I'd politely nod and say, "Yeah," but I was inwardly annoyed. My motivation for writing this book was to help you. I didn't believe I'd achieve a greater level of healing because my eating disorder behaviors had been few and far between for years.

Blessedly, I was wrong.

Psychological healing isn't linear. There isn't always a clear beginning or ending to this healing. The seed of healing is planted the day you first imagine what it would be like to be healthy or to no longer carry the pain or obsession, even if you continue to act on it for years after that thought. The day you tell someone you're struggling, you take that first step on the path to healing.

The growth that results from healing builds on itself, and like grief, there are layers to it. Just when you're certain you're fully healed, or you won't shed any more tears over a loss, another layer appears. Here is the beautiful part: the deeper the layer, the greater the effect of that healing on the rest of your life.

The year I spent writing this book was one of the most tumultuous of my life, and my healing was part of the reason for that tumult. My healing helped me walk away from a relationship that no longer served my highest good or my partner's. This involved moving out of a beautiful home and disconnecting from someone for whom I still held so much gratitude and love. It changed my social and financial circumstances, and it affected the hearts and lives of my children. It was a very good decision for all involved. And it was brutally sad.

Four months later, when my daughter became critically ill from the sudden onset of a chronic illness, the healing I'd done up to that point gave me the courage to ask for help from my community and to embrace its outpouring of love in all of its forms. Through my daughter's twenty-eight-day hospitalization, dozens of follow-up appointments, and a new job that had begun just one month before I ended my relationship, I called upon this community for support. And they showed up.

I grieved, I researched, I wrote. I held you in my heart and in my thoughts. I felt your pain, struggle, and frustration. It motivated me to keep writing. My writing grounded me, as it always does. I continued to cultivate my meditation practice. I reconnected with a spiritual teacher who helped me strengthen my intuition and remain focused on my purpose. I continued to heal.

The morning before our first draft was due to the publisher, I was again in a hospital room with my daughter. She'd been admitted the night before, and I'd hardly slept. It was still dark outside and the orange-yellow glow from the streetlights below was reflecting off the raindrops that ran down the window of our room. My daughter was asleep, and I was silently crying, spiraling downward into the emotional pit of despair, feeling alone and afraid.

I reached out to my spiritual teacher and asked for help. Even as I typed to her the news of Erin's hospitalization and a request for insight and help to get out of the spiral, there was a little niggling at the back of my mind telling me I had the tools to access that insight and climb out of the pit myself. I was just so tired. She sent loving words my way, told me she was in a rush to head out of town and would have to reconnect later in the day. She suggested I begin with breathing into the spiral.

I closed my eyes, took a deep breath, and immediately saw myself in an open field. It was raining and about thirty yards in front of me was a crowd of people holding black umbrellas. All I had to do was walk toward them. When I got to the group, they surrounded me, each one extending the hand that wasn't holding their umbrella. In each outstretched hand was a sphere of golden light reflecting a soft pink color. The light filled me from the top of my head down to my feet. I felt this message: *You're surrounded by help.*

This is what I want you to remember. Even when you're all alone, feeling like the end of this rough road is so far away that you can't even see it, you're surrounded by help. If you can't yet tell a friend or family member, start with books, podcasts, websites, or support groups. When one of those is out of reach, look for another. And when you're sitting alone in a dark room quietly crying, and you feel like there's no one you can talk to, close your eyes, and just focus on your breath. Do this for as long as it takes to feel your nervous system calm and your mind clear.

In the end, we're the ones who heal ourselves. We do this through our openness to the support available to us. We heal ourselves by doing the work. Peeling the layers back over and over and over. And we heal ourselves when we help each other.

Thank you for helping me heal. Thank you for holding one of the black umbrellas and being part of the light. I'm holding one for you, too.

Love,

Melissa

Book Club Study Questions

1. In what ways do you see diet culture manifesting today?
2. What generational differences did you see in Alayna and Melissa's two stories and perspectives?
3. How do Melissa's and Alayna's messages differ, and how do they align?
4. Many of the themes presented here contribute to struggles with negative body image, even for people who don't have eating disorders. Which underlying theme presented in *FULL* is most prevalent in your life?
5. Is there a belief you hold about your body, or an aspect of your body, that's clearly a result of diet culture? What would you get back if you were able to let go of that belief?
6. What misconceptions did you hold about eating disorders prior to reading *FULL*?
7. What small changes can you make to help mitigate the impact of diet culture in your sphere of influence?
8. Which of the guideposts will be most helpful to you?

Recommendations from Our Bookshelves

<u>Directly Related to Eating Disorders:</u>

Almost Anorexic: Is My (or My Loved One's) Relationship with Food a Problem? (The Almost Effect) by Jennifer J. Thomas, PhD, and Jenni Schaefer

Brain over Binge: Why I Was Bulimic, Why Conventional Therapy Didn't Work, and How I Recovered for Good by Kathryn Hansen

Eating in the Light of the Moon: How Women Can Transform Their Relationship with Food Through Myths, Metaphors, and Storytelling by Arika Rapson and Anita A. Johnston, PhD

Goodbye Ed, Hello Me: Recover from Your Eating Disorder and Fall in Love with Life by Jenni Schaefer

Life Without Ed: How One Woman Declared Independence from Her Eating Disorder and How You Can Too by Jenni Schaefer and Thom Rutledge

Intuitive Eating: A Revolutionary Anti-Diet Approach by RDN Evelyn Tribole, MS and RDN Elyse Resch, MS

The Intuitive Eating Workbook: Ten Principles for Nourishing a Healthy Relationship with Food by Evelyn Tribole, MS and Elyse Resch, MS

Skills-Building:

Atomic Habits: An Easy and Proven Way to Build Good Habits and Break Bad Ones by James Clear

Book of Forgiving: The Fourfold Path for Healing Ourselves and Our World by Desmond Tutu and Mpho Tutu

Building a Life Worth Living: A Memoir by Marsha M. Linehan

DBT Skills Training Manual by Marsha M. Linehan

The Dialectical Behavior Therapy Skills Workbook: Practical DBT Exercises for Learning Mindfulness, Interpersonal Effectiveness, Emotion Regulation & Distress Tolerance by Matthew McKay, PhD, Jeffrey C. Wood, and Jeffrey Brantley

Loving What Is: Four Questions That Can Change Your Life by Byron Katie and Stephen Mitchell

The Power of Attachment: How to Create Deep and Lasting Intimate Relationships by Diane Poole Heller, PhD

The Power of Habit: Why We Do What We Do in Life and Business by Charles Duhigg

Radical Acceptance by Tara Brach

Welcome Home: A Guide to Building a Home for Your Soul by Najwa Zebian

Personal Development:

The Courage to be Disliked by Ichiro Kishimi and Fumitake Koga

The Gifts of Imperfection by Brené Brown

I Thought It Was Just Me (but it isn't): Making the Journey from "What Will People Think?" to "I Am Enough" by Brené Brown

Pursuit of Perfect by Tal Ben-Shahar

Rising Strong by Brené Brown

The Seat of the Soul by Gary Zukav

Untamed by Glennon Doyle

The Untethered Soul by Michael A. Singer

The Way of Integrity: Finding the Path to Your True Self by Martha Beck

Acknowledgments

Alayna

My parents, Tom and Patty Burke, are my best friends. Mom, thank you for giving up your personal time to take me to every single doctor appointment, no matter what. Dad, thank you for remaining calm and sitting with me at my worst. Thank you both for believing that the true me was always there and for pulling me into a more beautiful life.

Nathan, thank you for being my earliest role model. You make me smile when no one else can, no matter how hard I try not to. I wouldn't be able to do this without you always cheering me on.

Melissa Kelley, there's no way I'd be writing this book at all if you hadn't jumped into this project full-heartedly (pun intended). You inspire me. Thank you for believing in this whole process and keeping me accountable.

Maddie Beerman, thank you for taking me out to breakfast one morning and telling me I should write a book. Here we are.

Shannon, my dietitian, thank you for being persistent with me. Even when I was a bitch at appointments, you never gave up on me. You led me to where I am today.

Thank you, Kari, my therapist, for teaching me what it means to be okay with taking up space. You taught me skills that I'll use for the rest of my life and skills that I share with others.

Audrey Dickherber, thank you for being the first friend to get me out of the house at my worst. You've always been the big sister I never had.

Uncle Mike, thank you for giving me advice on starting a book. Thank you for your endless support in all areas of my life.

Thank you, Jim Johnson and Incarnate Word Academy, for making my high school days doable. You taught me how to create balance in my life.

Thank you to everyone who has opened up to me on social media or in person about similar struggles. You've encouraged me to keep being vulnerable every day.

Finally, thank you to all of my friends from grade school, high school, and college. You each are a blessing in my life. There are countless friends that I'd like to name and thank. You all know who you are, and I love you. Thank you for supporting me.

Melissa

I'm eternally grateful to my parents, Bob and Barb Kelley, for finding and funding my treatment. This was a path none of us chose, and one with little light back in the 1980s. My healing journey was messy, and you're the reason I'm still here today.

Thank you, Alayna, Tom, and Patty Burke for bringing me into this project and making this book a reality. Each of you has played a significant role in my life, and I'm so grateful for your love and friendship.

Athena and Erin Kelley, you've been my greatest teachers, and I've made it to this level of healing because of you. Thank you for encouraging me to keep writing when I thought I was too tired or was feeling overwhelmed.

Thank you, Colleen Boschert, Amy Phillips, Erin Eberhard, Michael Kelley, and Meghan Pauly for always showing up. I think Rooster looks down on his Kelley Kids proudly.

Aunt Ces (Leslie Hardt), thank you for coming to group therapy in the middle of the week after a long work day (for months), for making the tough call to Mom and Dad in Europe to tell them I was sick again, and for being steadfast in your love and support of all the Kelley Kids. We hit the aunt jackpot!

Leah, Tina, Tammi, and Anne, thank you for your sisterhood in this healing. Each of you has been part of my growth and holds a special place in my heart.

Finally, thank you to all of the people over the years who've asked for my perspective on eating disorders. Most of you are loved ones of someone suffering from this disease, desperately seeking answers. Thoughts of your struggling daughters/friends and your desire to better understand them kept me going when this felt too hard. While I still don't have the answers you seek, I pray there's something in this book that speaks to you.

My greatest prayer for all of you is hope. Hope for a FULL life.

About the Authors

Alayna Burke started her idea for *FULL* as an eighteen-year-old senior in high school. She grew up in Saint Charles, Missouri, and always loved to write as a kid. Alayna developed anorexia, stemming from anxiety and depression, as a sixteen-year-old. Outpatient treatment and a strong support system helped Alayna recover in about two years, although the voice of her eating disorder still nags at her every once in a while. Alayna often wished there was a book out there from the voice of a teen who could relate to her, so she's providing just that for other women. *FULL* is Alayna's first published work. She is currently pursuing an undergraduate degree in nutrition and exercise physiology with a minor in psychology at the University of Missouri. Alayna plans to become a registered dietitian.

Melissa Kelley grew up in Saint Charles, Missouri, the third of six children. Her love for writing began in high school and blossomed in her forties when she began blogging and writing a memoir. *FULL* is her first published work.

Throughout her career, Melissa has worked in both corporate and civic non-profit organizations. She currently holds a leadership position in a company whose mission is to make the planet better through environmental sustainability services. In 2018, Melissa was named one of Saint Louis' Most Influential Businesswomen by the St. Louis Business Journal.

Melissa holds a Bachelor of Arts in psychology from Truman State University and a Master of Business Administration from Washington University in Saint Louis. She lives with her two children, Athena Robin Kelley and Erin Iris Christine Kelley, and their Cavapoo, Noah, in Saint Louis, Missouri.

Made in the USA
Las Vegas, NV
16 November 2022